Creating Empowering Environments for People with Dementia

This edited volume addresses the environments that exacerbate, exclude, and stigmatise those living with dementia to explore designs and processes that can optimise well-being and independence.

Featuring the voices and opinions of people with dementia, the chapters showcase individual homes, special dementia facilities, different forms of care homes, and public spaces, from landscape to urbanism, as examples of how to meet the needs and preferences of those living with dementia now. As a response to a recent Cochrane meta-analysis (2022) which highlighted the problems associated with using traditional, medically orientated evaluative methods for environmental design, this book demonstrates a range of research methods that can be used to inform and investigate good co-design of dementia-enabling environments. Furthermore, the book addresses cultural differences in people's needs and illustrates past, ongoing, and novel initiatives worldwide.

Ultimately, this timely volume focuses on person-centred design that enables empowerment, quality of life, health, and citizenship in people living with dementia. It will be of value to researchers, scholars, and postgraduate students studying gerontology, dementia specifically, and those involved with architecture and the built environment for societal benefit more broadly.

Kevin Charras is Director at the Living Lab Aging and Vulnerabilities, Department of Geriatrics, University Hospital of Rennes, France.

Eef Hogervorst is Professor of Biological Psychology and Director of Dementia Research, Loughborough University, UK.

Sarah Wallcook is a Researcher at The Stockholm Gerontology Research Centre and affiliated to the Care Research Group, Department of Social Work at Stockholm University, Sweden.

Saskia Kuliga is a Postdoctoral Researcher and PI at the German Centre for Neurodegenerative Diseases (DZNE), Germany, and affiliated with the Department of Nursing Science, Faculty of Health at the University of Witten/ Herdecke in Witten, Germany.

Bob Woods is Emeritus Professor of Clinical Psychology of Older People at Bangor University, UK, and former clinical psychologist specialising in dementia care.

Aging and Mental Health Research

Series Editor: Martin Orrell

In the 21st century, the world's aging population is growing more rapidly than ever before. This is driving the international research agenda to help older people live better for longer and to find the causes and cures for chronic diseases such as dementia. This series provides a forum for the rapidly expanding field by investigating the relationship between the aging process and mental health. It compares and contrasts scientific and service developments across a range of settings, including the mental changes associated with normal and abnormal or pathological aging, as well as the psychological and psychiatric problems of the aging population. The series encourages an integrated approach between biopsychosocial models and etiological factors to promote better strategies, therapies and services for older people. Creating a strong alliance between the theoretical, experimental and applied sciences, the series provides an original and dynamic focus, integrating the normal and abnormal aspects of mental health in aging so that theoretical issues can be set in the context of important new practical developments in this field.

In this series

New Developments in Dementia Prevention Research
State of the Art and Future Possibilities
Edited by Kate Irving, Eef Hogervorst, Deborah Oliveira and Miia Kivipelto

Loneliness and Social Isolation in Old Age
Correlates and Implications
Edited by André Hajek, Steffi G. Riedel-Heller and Hans-Helmut König

Creating Empowering Environments for People with Dementia
Addressing Inclusive Design from Homes to Cities
Edited by Kevin Charras, Eef Hogervorst, Sarah Wallcook, Saskia Kuliga and Bob Woods

For more information about the series, please visit: www.routledge.com/Aging-and-Mental-Health-Research/book-series/AMHR

Creating Empowering Environments for People with Dementia

Addressing Inclusive Design from Homes to Cities

Edited by
Kevin Charras, Eef Hogervorst,
Sarah Wallcook, Saskia Kuliga
and Bob Woods

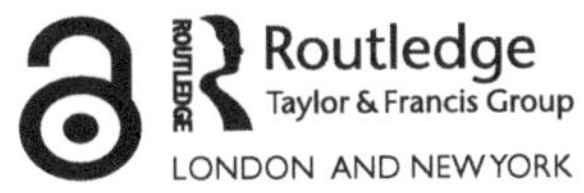

First published 2025
by Routledge
4 Park Square, Milton Park, Abingdon, Oxon OX14 4RN

and by Routledge
605 Third Avenue, New York, NY 10158

Routledge is an imprint of the Taylor & Francis Group, an informa business

British Library Cataloguing-in-Publication Data
A catalogue record for this book is available from the British Library

Library of Congress Cataloging-in-Publication Data
Names: Charras, Kevin, editor. | Hogervorst, Eef, editor. | Wallcook, Sarah, editor. | Kuliga, Saskia, editor. | Woods, Robert T., editor.
Title: Creating empowering environments for people with dementia : addressing inclusive design from homes to cities / edited by Kevin Charras, Eef Hogervorst, Sarah Wallcook, Saskia Kuliga, and Bob Woods.
Other titles: Aging and mental health research
Description: Abingdon, Oxon ; New York, NY : Routledge, 2025. | Series: Aging and mental health research | Includes bibliographical references and index.
Identifiers: LCCN 2024015526 (print) | LCCN 2024015527 (ebook) | ISBN 9781032543031 (hbk) | ISBN 9781032543024 (pbk) | ISBN 9781003416241 (ebk)
Subjects: MESH: Dementia | Built Environment
Classification: LCC RC523 .C74 2025 (print) | LCC RC523 (ebook) | NLM WT 155 | DDC 616.8/31—dc23/eng/20240516
LC record available at https://lccn.loc.gov/2024015526
LC ebook record available at https://lccn.loc.gov/2024015527

ISBN: 978-1-032-54303-1 (hbk)
ISBN: 978-1-032-54302-4 (pbk)
ISBN: 978-1-003-41624-1 (ebk)

DOI: 10.4324/9781003416241

Typeset in Sabon
by codeMantra

The electronic version of this book was funded to publish Open Access through Taylor & Francis' Pledge to Open, a collaborative funding open access books initiative. The full list of pledging institutions can be found on the Taylor & Francis Pledge to Open webpage.

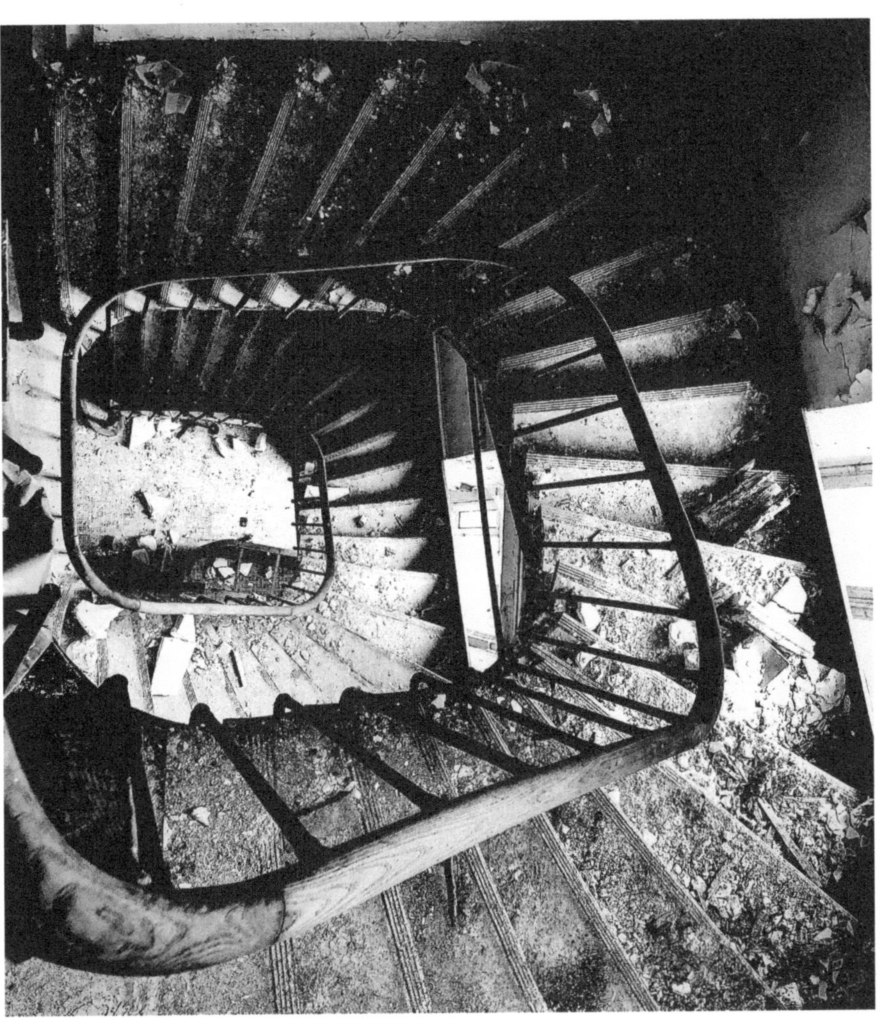

Figure 0.1 'Sanatorium' copyright Kevin Charras. A thought provoking illustration of how built environments designed to provide care for people have changed over time.

Contents

List of editors   *xiii*
List of contributors   *xvii*

Prologue: design for dementia: 50 years on   1
BOB WOODS

PART 1
**Setting the scene: history and underlying design
mainstreams and philosophies**   13

1   Use of theoretical models in dementia-inclusive design   15
MANISHA JAIN AND EEF HOGERVORST

2   Creating homes for individuals living with dementia:
the past, the present and the future   30
MARGARET CALKINS

3   Advances in research and practice on environmental design
of care facilities for people living with dementia   45
KEVIN CHARRAS

PART 2
People with dementia are central to the design process   55

4   The voice of people with dementia at the core
of environmental design   57
EMILY ONG, MARTIN ROBERTSON, DENNIS FROST,
HABIB CHAUDHURY AND RICHARD FLEMING

5   The use of virtual reality to support participatory design
    processes in environmental design for cognitive change   69
    LESLEY PALMER, MARTIN QUIRKE, JUNJIE HUANG
    AND JUDITH PHILLIPS

6   Improving housing decisions for and with people
    with dementia: a co-design approach   82
    JODI STURGE AND LOUISE MEIJERING

PART 3
Dementia friendly neighbourhoods   93

7   How can public organizations, transport systems and
    spaces be made more dementia friendly? Findings from
    participatory health research and architecture   95
    VERENA C. TATZER, BARBARA PICHLER, ELISABETH REITINGER,
    GESINE MARQUARDT AND KATHARINA HEIMERL

8   Rural and urban transportation and technology use:
    what needs to be considered?   109
    SARAH WALLCOOK, CAMILLA MALINOWSKY AND ANNA BRORSSON

9   Toilets: a key feature for inclusive design. Newbuild
    and refurbishment   119
    GILL MATHEWS, MARY MARSHALL AND HEATHER WILKINSON

10 Selected innovative research projects I   131
    10.1   *Project 1: dementia-enabling neighbourhoods –*
           participatory development of dementia-enabling
           neighbourhoods in Bremen 132
           JANISSA ALTONA, HENRIK WIEGELMANN, EMILY MENA,
           JULIA MISONOW, CHRISTOPH TEVES, BENJAMIN SCHÜZ
           AND KARIN WOLF-OSTERMANN
    10.2   *Project 2: inclusive co-research with people living*
           with dementia about wayfinding in their living
           environment and neighbourhood 137
           SASKIA KULIGA, MARTINA ROES AND JIM MANN

PART 4
General hospital design   **143**

11 Dementia-friendly hospitals: current state and future directions   145
SUZANNE TIMMONS AND EMMA O'SHEA

12 Architectural design guidance for general hospitals:
ways to implement proven concepts and to accommodate
future challenges   157
GESINE MARQUARDT AND KATHRIN BUETER

PART 5
Care home design   **169**

13 Translating environmental design knowledge into practice:
progress and challenges   171
RICHARD FLEMING AND JOHN ZEISEL

14 Sociotherapeutic living environments in long-term care
organisations   184
DEBBY GERRITSEN, HANNEKE NOORDAM,
HANNEKE NIJSTEN AND HANNEKE DONKERS

15 Dementia-friendly design: towards minimizing spatial
disorientation in residential care homes   195
ELENA CARBONE, LAURA MIOLA, ERIKA BORELLA
AND FRANCESCA PAZZAGLIA

16 Green care farms and other innovative settings   205
HILDE VERBEEK, INGEBORG PEDERSEN,
BRAM DE BOER AND SIMONE DE BRUIN

17 Selected innovative research projects II   216
    *17.1 Project 1: the German Environmental Audit
    Tool in nursing homes 217*
    ANNE FAHSOLD AND BERNHARD HOLLE

17.2 *Project 2: decision-making in care homes: the impact of the environment on people living with dementia sharing their everyday decisions 220*
RACHEL DALY

Epilogue 224
EEF HOGERVORST AND TRI BUDI RAHARDJO

Index 231

Editors

Kevin Charras is director of the Living Lab Aging and Vulnerabilities of the Geriatric Department at the University Hospital of Rennes (France). Kevin started his career as a psychologist in a psychiatric hospital before working for over 13 years as a head manager for the Fondation Médéric Alzheimer before creating the Living Lab in Rennes. His area of expertise focuses on environmental design (he collaborated with architects in over 60 nursing homes on this aspect) and psychosocial interventions for people living with dementia. He has authored and co-authored over 80 publications in scientific journals and has given talks at over 100 congresses internationally, as well as written professional reviews and academic books. He is also the author of a book on psychosocial interventions for people with dementia and co-author of three practical guides on caring for people with dementia through environmental and landscape design, technologies, and psychosocial interventions. Kevin Charras also teaches in universities in his areas of expertise and coordinates a degree in psychosocial interventions at the University of Caen (France).

Eef Hogervorst is Professor of Biological Psychology and Director of Dementia Research at Loughborough University, a top 10 University in the UK. Eef holds several visiting Professorial posts in the UK and Indonesia where she compares data of various cohorts on early diagnosis and primary, secondary, and tertiary prevention of dementia using lifestyle changes including exercise, nutrition, hormones, and design. She obtained over £10M funding for her research with collaborators and has published over 200 peer-reviewed international papers. This includes several books she edited and wrote chapters for, such as a state-of-the-art book within the same Taylor Francis series (commissioned by Prof Orrell) on prevention of dementia (2019) including world-renowned experts in this field (https://www.routledge.com/New-Developments-in-Dementia-Prevention-Research-State-of-the-Art-and-Future/Irving-Hogervorst-Oliveira-Kivipelto/p/book/9780367583200) as well as a Cambridge University commissioned state of the art book on hormones, cognition, and dementia after an expert conference on this topic organised by Eef at Loughborough (https://www.cambridge.org/core/books/hormones-cognition-and-dementia). Eef recently published an academic handbook for Routledge Taylor Francis with dementia specialist architects Professor Mike Riley and Bill Halsall (HLP) called *Design for Dementia: Living Well at Home* using the Loughborough and HLP evidence-based Chris and Sally home at BRE Watford as a case study https://www.amazon.co.uk/Design-Dementia-Living-Well-Home/dp/1032306483. As dementia expert, she consulted on Specialist Dementia Facilities for Leicestershire County Council and has provided similar consultancies in Singapore and Indonesia. Other chapters of books she was invited to contribute to include her research on dementia diagnostics, lifestyle, and dementia risk, as well as non-pharmacological interventions.

Sarah Wallcook is a researcher at The Stockholm Gerontology Research Centre and affiliated with the Care Research Group at the Department of Social Work, Stockholm University. Her current work focuses on developing co-research and collaborative models that support the development of social and environmental initiatives to support community-based health and participation in everyday life among older care-experienced people. Her doctoral thesis at the research group Cognitive Accessibility of Technology Use When Ageing at Home and in Society at the Division of Occupational Therapy, Karolinska Institutet, used multiple case studies and modern and traditional statistical methods to highlight the complex conditions of using everyday technology and its interplay in life outside home among people with and without dementia. Her doctoral studies were developed through her Marie Curie Early Career fellowship within the Interdisciplinary Network for Dementia Using Current Technology.

Saskia Kuliga currently is a postdoctoral researcher and PI at the German Centre for Neurodegenerative Diseases (DZNE), Site Witten, and affiliated with the University of Witten/Herdecke, and the ETH Zurich. She previously was a Postdoc Fellow with the German Academic Exchange Service (DAAD) at Singapore-ETH Centre Future Cities Laboratory Singapore, and with Information Science in Architecture at Bauhaus University Weimar. Her doctoral dissertation at the Center for Cognitive Science, within the trans-regional research centre Spatial Cognition DFG/SFB/TR8 focused on evaluating user experience and wayfinding behaviour in complex, architectural environments and building usability. She is a member of the German Society for Psychologists (DGPs), its subgroup Environmental Psychology, and the Environment and Dementia Special Interest Group Singapore. She has (co-)authored several academic publications in international peer-reviewed journals, conference proceedings, practice-oriented journals, and academic books.

Bob Woods is Emeritus Professor of Clinical Psychology with Older People at Bangor University. He studied Experimental Psychology at the University of Cambridge, before qualifying as a clinical psychologist at the University of Newcastle-upon-Tyne in 1975. He then worked for several years in the NHS in Newcastle, as a clinical psychologist with older people. Subsequently, he combined extensive clinical work with older people with academic appointments at the Institute of Psychiatry, London, and University College London. He was appointed the first Chair in Clinical Psychology with Older People in the UK, at Bangor University in 1996, and following his retirement in July 2017, he has been awarded the title Emeritus Professor. He was Director of the Dementia Services Development Centre Wales at Bangor University from its inception in 1999 until 2017. He has been closely involved with developments in dementia care in Wales through his role with the NHS Wales 1000 Lives plus quality improvement programme on dementia care. His research has focused on psychosocial approaches to working with people with dementia and their families. He has published widely, from research papers on dementia care and on depression in older people to textbooks for clinical psychologists to books for family carers and training packages.

Contributors

Janissa Altona, Henrik Wiegelmann, Emily Mena, Julia Misonow, and Christoph Teves are affiliated with the Institute of Public Health and Nursing Research (IPP) at the University of Bremen, Germany.

Margaret Calkins is affiliated with IDEAS Institute, Cleveland Heights, Ohio, USA.

Elena Carbone, Laura Miola, Erika Borella, and Francesca Pazzaglia are affiliated with the Department of General Psychology, University of Padova, Italy.

Habib Chaudhury is affiliated with the Department of Gerontology at Simon Fraser University, Vancouver, Canada.

Rachel Daly is affiliated with Dementia UK and University of Hertfordshire, UK.

Bram de Boer is affiliated with the Department of Health Sciences Research, Care and Public Health Research Institute, Maastricht University, Maastricht, The Netherlands.

Simone de Bruin is affiliated with Windesheim University of Applied Sciences, The Netherlands.

Anne Fahsold and Bernhard Holle are affiliated with the German Center for Neurodegenerative Diseases e.V. (DZNE), Site Witten, Germany as well as the Department of Nursing Science, Faculty of Health, University of Witten/Herdecke, Witten, Germany.

Richard Fleming is affiliated with the Faculty of Arts, Social Sciences and Humanities at the University of Wollongong, Australia.

Dennis Frost is dementia advocate and affiliated with Dementia Australia, within the Dementia Australia's Advisory Committee, Sydney, NSW, Australia, as well as the Dementia Friendly Kiama Advocacy Group, Kiama, NSW, Australia.

Katharina Heimerl is Associate Professor at the Department of Nursing Science, University of Vienna, Austria.

Junjie Huang and **Judith Phillips** are affiliated with the Faculty of Social Sciences, University of Stirling, Stirling, Scotland.

Manisha Jain is affiliated with the School of Sports Exercise and Health Sciences, NCSEM at Loughborough University, UK.

Camilla Malinowsky and **Anna Brorsson** are affiliated with the Division of Occupational Therapy, Department of Neurobiology, Care Sciences and Society at Karolinska Institutet, Sweden.

Jim Mann is dementia advocate and affiliated with the University of British Columbia, Vancouver, Canada.

Gesine Marquardt is Professor of Social and Health Care Buildings and Design at the Faculty of Architecture at the TUD Dresden University of Technology, Germany.

Kathrin Bueter is affiliated with the Faculty of Architecture, TUD Dresden University of Technology, and Chair for Social and Health Care Buildings and Design, Germany.

Gill Mathews, Mary Marshall, and **Heather Wilkinson** are affiliated with the University of Edinburgh and Hammond Care, for the UK and Europe.

Louise Meijering is affiliated with the Department of Demography, Faculty of Spatial Sciences at the University of Groningen, The Netherlands.

Hanneke Noordam is affiliated with Vilans.

Hanneke Nijsten, Hanneke Donkers and **Debby Gerritsen** are affiliated with the Department of Primary and Community Care, Radboud Institute for Health Sciences, Radboud Alzheimer Center, Radboud University Medical Center, Nijmegen, The Netherlands.

Emily Ong is dementia advocate in Singapore, at the Dementia Alliance International (DAI), TX, USA, within the Environmental Design Special Interest Group (ED-SiG).

Lesley Palmer and **Martin Quirke** are affiliated with the Dementia Services Development Centre at the University of Stirling, UK.

Ingeborg Pedersen is affiliated with the Department of Public Health Science, Faculty of Landscape and Society, Norwegian University of Life Sciences.

Barbara Pichler is affiliated with CAREWEB, Association for the Promotion of Societal Care Culture, Life, Old Age, Dementia and Dying, as well as the Department of Occupational Therapy, University of Applied Sciences Wiener Neustadt, Austria.

Tri Budi Rahardjo is affiliated with Universitas Respati in Yogyakarta and Jakarta, Indonesia.

Elisabeth Reitinger is Associate Professor at the Department of Nursing Science, University of Vienna, Austria.

Martina Roes is Site Speaker, Group Leader, and Professor at the German Center for Neurodegenerative Diseases e.V. (DZNE), Site Witten, Germany, as well as at the Department of Nursing Science, Faculty of Health, at the University of Witten/Herdecke, Witten, Germany.

Martin Robertson is dementia advocate and affiliated with "ECREDibles" at the Edinburgh Centre for Research on the Experience of Dementia, School of Health in Social Science, University of Edinburgh, Edinburgh, Scotland.

Benjamin Schüz and **Karin Wolf-Ostermann** are affiliated with the Institute of Public Health and Nursing Research (IPP), University of Bremen, Germany, and also with Health Sciences Bremen, Germany.

Jodi Sturge is affiliated with the Department of Design, Production and Management, Faculty of Engineering Technology, University of Twente, Enschede, The Netherlands.

Verena C. Tatzer is a postdoctoral researcher/teacher at the Department of Occupational Therapy at the University of Applied Sciences Wiener Neustadt, Austria.

Suzanne Timmons and **Emma O'Shea** are affiliated with the Centre for Gerontology & Rehabilitation, University College Cork, Ireland.

Hilde Verbeek is the chair of the Limburg Living Lab in Ageing and Long-Term Care and Professor of Long-Term Care Environments at the Department of Health Services Research, Care and Public Health Reseach Institute, Maastricht University, Maastricht in the Netherlands.

John Zeisel is founder of the I'm Still Here Foundation, Hopeful Aging R&D, and Hearthstone Alzheimer Care. He has authored "Inquiry by Design: Environment/Behavior/Neuroscience in Architecture, Interiors, Landscape, and Planning" and "I'm Still Here: A New Philosophy of Alzheimer Care." His mission is to change the public narrative of dementia from despair, disease, and drugs, to hope, disability, and ecopsychosocial treatment.

Prologue

Design for dementia: 50 years on

Bob Woods

A personal reflection

It is a pleasure to introduce this volume on behalf of my fellow editors, who have borne the greater part of the responsibility for its genesis and fruition. Design for dementia has fascinated me throughout my career as a practising clinical psychologist and dementia researcher so in introducing this volume I found myself looking back at my personal experiences and observations of dementia care environments and attempts at seeking to shape them.

My first exposure to a care environment for people living with dementia was in 1973. It was a 'psychogeriatric ward' in a large mental hospital, situated in the countryside a few miles outside the city. Between thirty and forty women received care on this ward, one of many in this hospital, built over 100 years previously. Patients slept in dormitories, with barely space between beds for a small locker. There was no privacy, few if any personal possessions, and even items of clothing were shared. A single large open plan day-room, with a high ceiling, featured lines of armchairs and an area with small dining tables and chairs. The care environment was **institutional**, with a rigid routine and 'batch nursing' was the order of the day. Patients were got up, dressed, toileted, fed, washed and put to bed in batches, according to the staff timetable and availability rather than individual needs or preferences.

As I discovered subsequently, in many ways this ward was typical in the UK in the 1970s, but, fortuitously, it was remarkable in that it was part of a project to transform the therapeutic environment in various parts of this former asylum, a project that empowered staff to examine care practice and make changes. In small ways, this enabled staff to break free from the constraints of the rigid routine and spend time interacting with patients and attending to individual needs (Savage & Widdowson, 1974). Previously the care regime had increased patients' dependency, but this example of 'milieu therapy' led to ward staff reporting 'that patients were more responsive to their environment and less incontinent' (Woods & Britton, 1977, p. 107). Thus, my memories of that first experience are not simply frustration and anger prompted by a grim institutional environment, but, much more

DOI: 10.4324/9781003416241-1

optimistically, of the small changes to the physical and social environment that could make a difference to the lives of people living with dementia. Of the husband of a woman in her 50s with young onset dementia visiting daily, and the staff putting on music so they could dance together; of the doors from the day-room to the outside gardens being finally opened, so staff could take patients out for walks to see and smell the flowers and enjoy the fresh air; of patients getting up and having breakfast when they were ready, not when routine demanded. Most importantly, it was evident that changes to the **social environment** did not need to wait for the **physical environment** to change, desirable as that may be.

As the 1970s progressed, I discovered that in many parts of the UK, the physical environment for dementia care was already changing, with a divergence evident between the long-term care provided by the National Health Service (NHS), in hospital settings no longer fit for purpose, and exciting developments in care homes provided by local authorities (what is now described as 'social care'). These residential homes were moving on from the legacy of workhouse provision inherited in 1948 (see Townsend, 1962), with purpose-built homes situated in local communities becoming the norm. There was debate, however, as to where provision for people with dementia fitted in these developments. In some areas, such as Newcastle-upon-Tyne, where I trained and worked until 1980, specialist homes with the unfortunate label of homes for the 'elderly mentally infirm' (or EMI homes) were established, catering mainly for people with dementia. While the positive view of this development was that these homes could develop skills and expertise in meeting the needs of residents with dementia, there was a view that in so doing people with dementia were undergoing **segregation and** would be better served through **integration** with their peers who were not experiencing cognitive impairment. Even where there were no specialist homes, segregation still occurred through the creation of special units within homes. There was the potential for stigma and rejection of the cognitively impaired by those more able, perhaps wishing to distance themselves from a feared future.

Also at this time, there were moves to reduce the **institutional** elements of residential care homes by establishing small living groups (of 8–10 residents) within care homes, making for a more **homely** care environment, where residents could be more engaged in day-to-day activities, including serving food and sharing meals, with a small kitchen provided for each group. Seating areas offered small clusters of armchairs, enhancing opportunities for social interaction in contrast with the traditional side-by-side around the walls chair arrangement seen in institutional settings (Woods & Britton, 1985, p. 219). There was debate regarding what proportion of people with dementia could be included in a small living group for it to be viable, but in an early evaluation in Newcastle we found an increase in life satisfaction and engagement amongst residents following the introduction of group living in a non-specialist residential home, where many of the residents had mild or moderate dementia (Rothwell et al., 1983).

The early 1980s saw great progress in the trialling and implementation of psychosocial approaches for people with dementia – notably Reality Orientation (RO) and reminiscence approaches began to be widely used in many care settings for people with dementia; '24-hour RO' had clear implications for environmental design as well as care practice, with studies showing the value of **orientation aids** such as signposting and information boards in hospitals and care homes. These were described as contributing to a 'prosthetic environment', compensating for dementia-related disability (e.g. Holden & Woods, 1982, pp. 25–26). Working now in London, I had an opportunity to visit and work with care facilities in several different areas and saw examples of new homes heavily and explicitly influenced by RO concepts. More dramatically, examples of **reminiscence**-based environmental design also began to appear, in hospital settings as well as care homes, with rooms decorated, furnished and equipped in a style thought to reflect a period much earlier in the life of the person with dementia. Reminiscence would then take place not just as part of a structured group, but informally with the use of the many different memory triggers across multiple senses providing a rich basis for social interaction, sharing of memories and of stories from the past.

The future shape of dementia care provision was subject to broader forces as the 1980s progressed. There was a move to close the large 19th century mental hospitals and to ultimately replace them with 'community care'. Partly driven by scandals regarding poor quality care, services for people with learning disabilities were at the vanguard of this movement. Principles of '**normalisation**' underpinned these developments, with the vision being to provide care and support in ordinary housing within the community. In relation to dementia, an influential report was published by the King's Fund (1986) setting out an approach based on the **rights** of the person with dementia, and the need to combat devaluation and depersonalisation of the person with dementia. At this time, there was much questioning whether it was desirable or necessary at all to have institutions providing care for older people and for people with dementia. Were the manifold problems associated with institutional care, such as apathy, dependence and social withdrawal, an inevitable result of communal living, rather than examples of poor practice? Could the quality of care be improved?

As it happened, the closure of the large mental hospitals provided an opportunity for a fresh approach to design of care facilities. Around London in the late 1980s and early 1990s, additional funding was made available to establish new facilities to house the remaining residents of the hospitals (many of whom had a moderate to severe degree of dementia) closer to the communities from where they had come. Although, still recognisable as care homes, the new facilities were generally built to a smaller scale with smaller living units, resulting in more favourable staff-resident staffing ratios than had been the case in the traditional hospital wards. As part of this movement, the **'domus philosophy'** was expounded (see Woods, 1996, p. 374), aiming *inter alia* to correct the avoidable and accommodate the unavoidable consequences of dementia. Residents were encouraged to have an active role, maintaining independence and preserved abilities, with the living unit on a domestic scale, and precedence was given to psychological and emotional aspects of care. Needs of staff were considered alongside those of residents, their role being paramount in maintaining the quality of care. Evaluations suggested that levels of activity and interaction increased in homes designed on these principles, and those of us directly involved in the transfer of people with dementia from the traditional hospital wards to these new, homely settings witnessed changes that were a dramatic confirmation of the impact the environment can have on people with dementia. We were aware, of course, that similar small-scale, homely units were being established internationally, such as 'cantou' in France and 'group-living' in Sweden (see Woods, 1996, pp. 373–377), although we felt frustrated at the compromises that appeared to be necessary to meet UK legal requirements. For example, making the kitchen the hub of the home and involving residents fully in the preparation of meals was difficult to achieve, despite being a core aspect of 'home'.

What did emerge clearly from this process was the positive impact on the families of the residents with dementia of the move from the large, often inaccessible, institutions to the new homely environments in their own locality. It was possible for family members, if they wished, to be much more involved in the day-to-day care of their relative, and to maintain engagement with them. Guilt feelings were reduced, and family members adopted a variety of roles, some spouses spending much of their days with their relative (Woods & Macmillan, 1994). There was a new challenge for homes, of course, in how best to support **family involvement**. More involvement led to greater scrutiny and the need for more effective communication than had been thought necessary previously.

As the NHS steadily reduced the extent of its provision for long-term care of people with dementia in the UK in the 1990s, the independent sector was encouraged to grow to meet the gap. This included not-for-profit homes, run by charities, as well as the private sector. One of the homes I had helped establish in South London was run by a leading charity for the welfare of older people, and in 1995 I was approached by another charity to assist with an evaluation of staff training and development at a new purpose-built home they had established just outside London. By good fortune, this gave me the opportunity to collaborate with Tom Kitwood, from Bradford University, who had been charged with delivering the initial training for the staff of the new home. It was at this time that Kitwood's writing and teaching regarding person-centred care and the social psychological influences on the development and progression of dementia were beginning to change the language and landscape of dementia care provision. The combination of a new home, which won architectural awards for its design, and training from the leading figure in dementia care seemed an irresistible combination. However, detailed observation of the experience of residents with dementia, using the Dementia Care Mapping observational tool developed by Kitwood, suggested there was substantial room for improvement, and organisational changes proved to be needed before improvements in residents' well-being and quality of life were observed (Lintern et al., 2002). The **interaction between physical environment and social environment** again proved complex, and it was evident that the social environment was influenced not just by the attitudes, skills and knowledge of the staff providing care, but also by the organisational systems in place, which could detract from high-quality care (Woods, 2019).

The increased role of the independent sector in dementia care led to many providers across the UK looking at upgrading an existing care environment to be suitable for people with dementia-related needs, in addition to those seeking to build a new facility. Fortunately for those of us called in to advise on these developments, a number of **design checklists** were available by the late 1990s which could be used as a basis for consultation (see, e.g. Day et al., 2000 and the many helpful publications from the Dementia Services Development Centre at Stirling University). These emphasised, for example, the small size of units; domestic, familiar and homely (i.e. non-institutional) design; compensating for disability, providing an understandable, orientating environment and maximising independence; single rooms and plenty of space for personal possessions; secure outdoor areas; privacy; and building in safety features unobtrusively. Although there was a general lack of empirical evidence, these recommendations enjoyed a consensus of expert opinion. In seeking to assist care providers in North Wales (where I was now based), it became clear that applying these principles to existing homes presented many challenges and required many compromises, balancing one principle against another, especially where the home had originally been a grand house, with numerous corridors, staircases and annexes. New-build homes appeared easier, with compromises required largely due to funding issues and particular features of the site for the home. The resulting homes were certainly a world apart from my first experience of dementia care, and gratifyingly engaged with families from the outset (Hughes et al., 2019). However, it was always apparent that despite single, en-suite rooms, personalisation, wonderful views, easy access to gardens and social engagement with friends and families, lapses in care quality could occur where staff were not provided with the support and resources to maintain person-centred care.

Having withdrawn almost completely from long-term care of people with dementia, in the late 2000s the NHS found that a significant proportion of its acute **general hospital** beds were occupied by people with dementia and reports emerged (e.g. from the Alzheimer's Society) that were highly critical of the quality of care provided in these settings. In Wales, the Older People's Commissioner (2011) recommended simple and responsive changes to the physical environment to improve matters, pointing to resources such as 'Enhancing the healing Environment' (King's Fund, 2009). One of the aims was to reduce the disorientating and potentially frightening effects of admission to hospital for people with dementia, by use of clear signage, use of colour and clearer access to toilet facilities. This complemented major projects at local, regional and national levels to improve the awareness, skills and attitudes of all staff working in general hospitals and to identify more readily those affected by dementia and their specific needs, which formed a major preoccupation in the last few years of my professional career.

Why this volume?

Other contributions in this volume will provide a fuller account and overview of the relevant background and history of this field, but my personal journey persuades me of the need for this volume. We cannot ignore the scale of the challenge associated with dementia. The number of people affected by dementia continues to grow around the world. Alzheimer's Disease International (ADI) estimated that there were over 55 million people worldwide living with dementia in 2020 with an anticipated 78 million in 2030 and 139 million in 2050 (ADI, 2024). This is before considering the even greater numbers – typically family and friends – who provide care and support for those with a dementia. In addition to the human costs, the economic costs are staggering: ADI (2024) estimates the annual global cost of dementia is more than US$ 1.3 trillion rising to US$ 2.8 trillion by 2030 and points out that if global dementia care were a country, it would be the 14th largest economy in the world!

It is in this context that attention is needed as to how best to design environments and facilities that support and enable people living with dementia to have the best possible quality of life. This will involve supporting meaningful independent activities, including everyday activities, but also leisure and travel, to optimise well-being, dignity and independence. Many guidelines have already been written on dementia design, both for lay-people and design professionals, including the 2020 World Alzheimer Report 'Design, dignity, dementia: dementia-related design and the built environment' (ADI, 2020). What the current volume sets out to do is to bring together world-renowned researchers in this area alongside the voices of people with dementia to discuss inclusive dementia design of the environment in the public realm. The philosophy underlying the book focuses on person-centred design, with its emphasis on respect, dignity and working together to empower and enable citizenship in people living with dementia.

The book provides a historical review of design that works to support independence for people living with dementia, but also gives an overview of ongoing novel projects and a view to future developments including both established and junior researchers working in this field. It will provide new entrants to the field, as well as those with an established interest, with an overview of the state of the art, to be able to see the areas where consensus has been reached and, as importantly, those areas requiring more thought and further exploration. It showcases examples of best practice in environmental design, both in services specifically for people with dementia and in facilities for the general population, where design enables buildings and services to be accessible for those with dementia. With support from an INTER-DEM (the pan-European research network on psychosocial approaches in dementia https://interdem.org/) task force, the book addresses cultural differences in needs and illustrates ongoing and novel European and East Asian initiatives in this area.

The application of the available knowledge has, at best, been patchy. There are still many examples of poor design for people living with dementia. Indeed, there are many areas, including a high proportion of National Dementia Plans, where there is little or no awareness of the knowledge of how to design well for people living with dementia. This book explores the knowledge to practice divide and how it is being overcome.

The structure of the volume

In January 2022, the team started work on this book with interested INTER-DEM experts after several online meetings. This book was very much supported by excellent post-docs Sarah Wallcook and Saskia Kuliga as well as the senior input from eminent experts such as Professor Richard Fleming.

The contributions fall into five main sections. The first, Part 1, sets the scene, introducing both the history of the field and the underlying philosophies and theoretical perspectives. Thus, Jain and Hogervorst elaborate on the medical model, setting out the diversity of conditions included under the umbrella term 'dementia', their variability over time and between people and the powerful influence of other conditions, leading to a requirement for person-centred design. Calkins provides an overview of the development of the field, from the perspective of one of the leading figures in the design of care facilities, whilst Charras sets out important theoretical perspectives and considers the need for appropriate research designs in this field.

The second section, Part 2, focuses on a key theme for this volume: the inclusion of people with dementia at the heart of the design process. Ong et al. provide a context for this endeavour and provide examples of how this has been achieved. Palmer et al. show how virtual reality offers promise in enabling people with dementia to make the most effective input to design, providing feedback on their experience of a design before any bricks are laid! Sturge and Meijering provide a further example of a co-design process, in this case in relation to designing conversation starters to support decision-making. It should be noted that throughout the volume further examples may be found of the inclusion of people with dementia in the design process.

Part 3 examines dementia-friendly neighbourhoods. Tatzer et al. provide a wide-ranging contribution, including public buildings such as museums and libraries, public spaces and transportation. Wallcook et al. also examine transportation, here focusing on the way in which technology can be a barrier to transport use if not carefully designed. Mathews et al. tackle the important but often overlooked topic of provision of toilets in public places, and the impact this has on people with dementia. This section is completed by two brief contributions from early-career researchers (Altona et al., and Kuliga et al.), focusing on wayfinding in urban environments, using a variety of innovative research methods.

Design issues in general hospitals are the theme of Part 4, with important contributions from Timmons and O'Shea and from Marquardt and Bueter that cover a range of design issues, including consideration of Emergency Departments, where too often people with dementia have difficult experiences.

Part 5 is focused on the design of care facilities, probably the most established domain in the field. Fleming and Zeisel, who have contributed so much to this field over many years, provide an important contribution, addressing the implementation gap and detailing some of various ways they and others have sought to reduce this. Gerritsen et al. examine the potential benefits of grouping residents in care homes according to psychosocial needs, whilst Carbone et al. look at navigability within care home settings. Verbeek et al. discuss innovative alternatives to conventional care homes, including green care farms and dementia villages, which have attracted much interest in recent years. The section is completed by two further contributions from early-career researchers: Fahsold & Holle describe the adaptation of an environmental audit tool, while Daly discusses the impact of the environment on the decision-making of people with dementia in care homes.

In the final chapter of the book Hogervorst and Rahardjo present an account of selected examples of person-based approaches across a number of countries, including Eef Hogervorst's personal experience of how the physical and social environment do not always work together for the benefit of people living with dementia. A heart-felt plea for a truly person-centred approach, backed up by appropriate funding and valuing of all involved provides a fitting conclusion to the volume.

A personal reflection revisited

Fifty years on, to what extent has progress been made? Positive change is evident, but caveats remain. I am struck by how many of the themes that have been apparent over the years are still relevant today, with a number addressed specifically in this volume.

- Improving **general hospital** ward (and Emergency Department) design (see Part 4 of this book) can be seen as one aspect of working towards a dementia-friendly community, where all mainstream facilities are welcoming and accessible to people living with dementia, unthought of 50 years ago. However, given the proportion of people with dementia using these facilities, it is amazing that it took so long to realise the need – far from being dementia-friendly, too many hospitals were dementia-blind.

- Care homes (see Calkins, this volume and Part 5) are, by and large, much more **homely** and less **institutional** in design. In general, though, in the UK at least, the notion of ordinary living, supported in ordinary housing in the community, arising from '**normalisation**' principles, seems a lost cause, with ever larger facilities being built, justified on the grounds of cost. My understanding is that a number of original '**domus philosophy**' homes are no longer operational (including the one I helped to design!) – they were judged to be too expensive, due in part to their small-scale nature. This could be interpreted as indicating that as a society we are not prepared to pay the costs of this exemplary type of care for people living with dementia.

- **Family involvement** has come to the fore once again in recent years, with a campaign being needed in the UK to guarantee family access to care homes as partners in care, not simply as 'visitors', an optional extra to be dismissed when inconvenient. Sadly, many families were not able to be with their loved ones during the pandemic because of rulings that did not take into account the importance of their input. Arguably, it is loss of trust and poor communication with families that underlies many of the scandals in care quality that continue to surface.

- The human **rights** of people with dementia (including the right to family life) are discussed much more openly these days (see Charras, this volume), often refreshingly by people with dementia themselves, but challenges remain in advanced dementia to ensure these rights are respected, especially in communal living settings.

- The debate regarding **segregation vs. integration** has moved on but is still alive, to the extent that people with dementia find themselves excluded from activities and services. The concern now is to offer people with dementia **inclusion,** both in the use of facilities and services, but also, importantly, in the whole process of design and evaluation (see Ong et al., this volume). We see whole dementia villages being established (see Verbeek et al., this volume), with everything the person needs on the same campus. For example, is it preferable to have a hairdressing salon/shop/café/health clinic, etc., within your care home (used only by people with dementia), rather than continue to use the mainstream facilities within the community? Does this detract from encouraging community facilities (including leisure centres, libraries, primary care centres, shopping malls) taking steps to become dementia friendly (see Part 3)?

- Finally, the need to understand the **interaction between the physical environment** and the **social environment** remains pressing. Care facilities may be more homely, but the scope for lapses in care quality remains. The design of the care system involves leadership, organisation, shared values, staff support, positive attitudes, and a physical environment that supports the social environment created. Aspects of the physical environment can misfire if the social environment is not in tune: **orientation aids** (see Carbone et al., this volume) may be poorly designed or inaccurate; camouflaging exits and other hazards or the use of trompe l'oeil may be seen as deceiving the person with dementia; **reminiscence** features may reflect the wrong period of the person's life, or be associated with an unhappy memory, or if immersive may again be seen as an act of deception. **Design check-lists** (see Part 5) have their use, but some caution is needed: one of the most positive dementia care environments I have personally visited, in New York at the invitation of dementia design champion John Zeisel, would have actually fared badly in some respects. It had long corridors, no outside space and shared bedrooms, but appeared to be a wonderful living environment, due to the very positive social environment supported by the staff. Check-lists and environmental audits have their place but may not always capture the essence of person-centred care, when the physical and social environments combine to support the individual, with a unique biography and profile of needs and preferences.

References

Alzheimer's Disease International (2020). *Design, dignity, dementia: Dementia-related design and the built environment.* World Alzheimer Report 2020. https://www.alzint.org/resource/world-alzheimer-report-2020/ Accessed 01/02/2024.

Alzheimer's Disease International (2024). *Dementia statistics.* https://www.alzint.org/about/dementia-facts-figures/dementia-statistics/ Accessed 01/02/2024.

Day, K., Carreon, D. & Stump, C. (2000). The therapeutic design of environments for people with dementia: a review of the empirical research. *Gerontologist, 40*(4), 397–416.

Holden, U.P. & Woods, R.T. (1982). *Reality orientation: psychological approaches to the 'confused' elderly.* Edinburgh: Churchill Livingstone.

Hughes, S., Woods, B., Algar-Skaife, K., Jelley, H. & Jones, C.H. (2019). A collaborative approach: care staff and families working together to safeguard the quality of life of residents living with advanced dementia. *Journal of Central Nervous System Disease, 11*, 1–9. https://doi.org/10.1177/1179573519843872

King's Fund (1986). *Living well into old age: applying principles of good practice to services for people with dementia.* London: King's Fund.

King's Fund (2009). *Enhancing the healing environment: a guide for NHS trusts.* London: King's Fund.

Lintern, T., Woods, B. & Phair, L. (2002). Before and after training: a case study of intervention. In S. Benson (Ed.), *Dementia topics for the Millennium and beyond* (pp. 106–112). London: Hawker.

Older People's Commissioner for Wales (2011). *Dignified care? The experiences of older people in hospital in Wales.* https://olderpeople.wales/wp-content/uploads/2022/05/Dignified-Care-Full-Report.pdf Accessed 23/04/2024.

Rothwell, N.A., Britton, P.G. & Woods, R.T. (1983). The effects of group living in a residential home for the elderly. *British Journal of Social Work, 13,* 639–643.

Savage, B. & Widdowson, T. (1974). Revising the use of nursing resources. *Nursing Times, 70,* 1372–1374, 1424–1427.

Townsend, P. (1962). *The last refuge.* London: Routledge & Kegan Paul.

Woods, R.T. (1996). Institutional care. In R.T. Woods (Ed.), *Handbook of the clinical psychology of ageing* (pp. 369–387). Chichester: Wiley.

Woods, B. (2019). Commentary on 'The caring organization' by Tom Kitwood. In T. Kitwood & D. Brooker (Eds.), *Dementia reconsidered, revisited: the person still comes first* (pp. 137–142). London: Open University Press.

Woods, R.T. & Britton, P.G. (1977). Psychological approaches to the treatment of the elderly. *Age & Ageing, 6,* 104–112.

Woods, R.T. & Britton, P.G. (1985). *Clinical psychology with the elderly.* Beckenham: Croom Helm/Chapman Hall.

Woods, R.T. & Macmillan, M. (1994). Home at last? Impact of a local 'homely' unit for dementia sufferers on their relatives. In D. Challis, B. Davies & K. Traske (Eds.), *Community care: new agendas and challenges from the UK and overseas* (pp. 75–85). Aldershot: Ashgate Publishing.

Part 1

Setting the scene: history and underlying design mainstreams and philosophies

Use of theoretical models in dementia-inclusive design

Manisha Jain and Eef Hogervorst

The traditional medical model and dementia as a disease with characteristic pathology

The increase in number of people living with dementia and its huge growing human and economic costs identifies this as an important worldwide issue (Alzheimer's Association, 2020). The traditional medical model describes functional changes seen in dementia and emphasises how these cognitive, sensorimotor and behavioural aspects affect activities in daily life, resulting in increasing dependency over time. These changes impact on specific design needs of the environments to better support care, quality of life and independence. The medical model has its foundation in describing dementia as a pathological condition, for which ultimately a clinical pharmaceutical solution will be found. However, to date, despite medical advances, there is no long-term cost-effective pharmacological cure, and the focus remains on the prevention of dementia. Prevention is described as (i) primary: before onset of symptoms; (ii) secondary: in the prodromal phases of dementia and (iii) tertiary: to prevent progression in dementia and to optimise independence (Irving et al., 2018).

Cost-effective and sustainable design should thus ideally promote independence and prevent functional decline. The medical model has its basis in the identification of brain pathology, using brain scans and biomarkers and its clinical counterparts, in terms of cognitive and behavioural deficits which impact on independence in activities of daily life. The model also assumes separate and clear categorisation of dementia sub-types, which may impact on different design needs. The different sub-types of dementia, their pathology and clinical manifestation with potential impact on design are described as follows.

Alzheimer's disease

The official link between brain pathology and particular behaviours was made in 1906 by Alois Alzheimer who described a rare case with early onset dementia, Augusta D (Hippius and Neundörfer, 2003). At the age of 50 in

DOI: 10.4324/9781003416241-3

1901, Augusta D presented with confusion, sleep and memory impairments and typical behavioural and psychological symptoms of dementia, such as paranoid delusions and aggression, which led to her hospitalisation by her husband. Her brain at post-mortem examination showed the distinctive fatty plaques and tangles in brain tissue under the microscope that we now associate with Alzheimer's disease (AD), the most common form of dementia. Her type of dementia, despite being used as a hallmark case to illustrate AD, is actually quite rare, as it is an early form (before the age of 65, which was termed as 'presenile' in the past), which usually has a strong genetic component (Wingo et al., 2012; Ayodele et al., 2021).

The post-mortem confirmation using the CERAD criteria for AD pathology is when, according to the older diagnostic criteria, a definite AD diagnosis can be made (McKhann et al., 1984). However, this AD pathology can also be found in people who have not shown signs of dementia during their lifetime (Jack et al., 2011). In Oxford, we examined post-mortem confirmed dementia using probable CERAD Alzheimer's pathology criteria (Hogervorst et al., 2003). We found that 42% of all dementia cases had pure AD pathology (n=71) and only 6.5% (n=11) had pure vascular dementia pathology (who had been diagnosed as CERAD negative). The other dementia cases all showed mixed brain pathologies at death. AD pathology is found in around 60–80% of dementia cases (Alzheimer's Association, 2020) and we do not often find dementia without this type of pathology at post-mortem. However, of 35 controls, eight were diagnosed as CERAD possible AD. So, in 23% of controls examined at first assessment, when the diagnoses of dementia had not been made, AD pathology was present. As this type of dementia often presents with memory and disorientation (in time, place, etc.) in the first instance, prompter aids in the house can help.

Vascular dementia

Vascular dementia, the second most common dementia, has a more stepwise progression with each strategic infarct, multiple smaller infarcts, or more extensive deep white matter disease (Wiederkehr et al., 2008; Hogervorst et al., 2003). As such, having a stroke is a major risk factor for dementia. This type of pathology is found by itself in only 5–10% of people with dementia and mixed pathology (e.g. with AD) is much more common (Hogervorst et al., 2003). Depending on where pathology initially presents, disinhibition and planning and/or language (e.g. naming) can be affected in the first instance (with anterior lesions), only later to be followed by memory problems. Support in the stepwise execution of instrumental activities of daily life tasks (dressing, cooking, etc.) can be done using technology (voice overs activated when timed cupboard doors open, etc.) and by supporting carers.

Importantly, all cardiovascular disease risk factors are risk factors for Alzheimer's disease and vascular dementia. Lifestyle changes (exercise, a healthy diet, not smoking), medication (to lower blood pressure and blood lipids, such as total cholesterol, and regulate diabetes) and other modifiable factors (e.g. head injury, lack of psychosocial activities, hearing loss) can help to reduce dementia by up to 40% according to a meta-analysis commissioned by the Lancet on the prevention of dementia (Livingston et al., 2020).

These factors are all also associated with poor cognitive performance in people who do not necessarily develop dementia in life. These modifiable factors also often cluster together with having low socioeconomic status, including having had little education and no financial means to support healthy lifestyles, including good diets, medical care and living in non-polluted, green environments with little stress (Irving et al., 2018; Wang et al., 2023).

Lewy body disease, Parkinson's dementia and frontotemporal dementia

Lewy body dementia was not initially taught as a separate dementia in medical schools, but in the mid-nineties its diagnostic clinical criteria were written up by McKeith et al. (1996). These were relatively recently revised to dementia with Lewy bodies, which included medical biomarkers (McKeith et al., 2017). This is the third most commonly occurring form of dementia, seen in about 25% of all dementia cases, where Parkinson's disease features follow cognitive impairments, such as planning and word finding issues, and other specific symptoms, such as disordered REM sleep and very vivid usually visual hallucinations, which are often only later followed by memory impairments. These hallucinations can be triggered by patterns in soft furnishings, wall and other decorations, for instance. Hallucinations including auditory or sensory forms (which are brain-generated stimuli perceived as having their origin in the outside world), can also occur in other types of dementia, defined as Behavioural and Psychological Symptoms associated with Dementia (BPSD). Again, mixed pathology (with AD or VaD) is common and results in worse dementia severity (Menšíková et al., 2022).

Other forms of dementia include frontotemporal dementia, which is characterised by planning and other cognitive issues, also later followed by memory impairments (APA, 1994). This manifestation is relatively rare (only in 5% of all dementia cases), but may sometimes be misdiagnosed as psychiatric disorders, due to lack of inhibition and other BPSD. When we did dementia research in Indonesia around 2010 (Hogervorst et al., 2011), frontotemporal or Lewy body dementia were not identified as separate types of dementia by the local psychiatrists. It was unclear whether these did not exist or were not recognised, in the case of Lewy body dementia as separate, for instance, from Parkinson's disease with dementia, where the motor and other Parkinsonian features come first and are then later followed by cognitive impairments (Emre et al., 2007). Both these types of dementia are characterised by Lewy body pathology (National Institute on Aging or NIA, 2021; Menšíková et al., 2022). Diagnosing this type of dementia is important as anti-psychotics are often given to calm the behavioural and psychological symptoms associated with dementia, but this can make Lewy body dementia much worse (NIA, 2021).

The need for a personalised description of the dementia journey: the impact of culture

As previously mentioned, our research at Oxford University using post-mortem confirmed dementia, showed that in most dementia cases at death mixed pathology was more common, rather than people presenting with either Alzheimer's, Lewy body or vascular pathologies alone (Hogervorst et al., 2003). It may be more important to obtain insight in the individual pathway of progression to dependency to respond with design alterations and the required specific environmental refurbishments. This assessment requires a personalised approach and knowledge of the individual, their prior functional abilities, needs and preferences.

This becomes apparent, for instance, as one of the criteria (e.g. in one of the most used diagnostic manuals, APA, 1994) to diagnose dementia according to consensus-based criteria, is that the symptoms should affect activities of daily life, such as cooking and shopping. In some countries and cultures, where for instance, men did not engage in such activities, adjustments should be made to the scales assessing dependency (Arifin and Hogervorst, 2015). Conversely, we found that women often had obtained less education in low-income, rural areas (Hogervorst et al., 2011). Adjustments should be made for educational levels, especially for some of the commonly used cognitive screening tests (e.g. the Mini Mental State Examination or MMSE). This was not always done in studies, perhaps leading to a very high dementia prevalence reported, particularly in women in low and middle-income countries or LMIC (Jain and Hogervorst, in preparation). Culture sensitive tests and lack of experience of exposure to testing and examination-like situations could further induce poor performance not reflective of people's actual abilities. So, cultural/educational appropriate and sensitive testing of the ability to function independently, rather than focus on disability, should be the focus of dementia screening assessments required to optimise the environment to live independently.

Progression of dementia symptoms to dependency: the influence of reserve capacity

While accumulation of different pathologies can lead to dementia, the combined pathological load can be offset by brain reserve (reflecting functional connections between brain cells) and/or cognitive reserve (reflecting cognitive coping skills, such as having more vocabulary, alternative problem-solving, etc., to mitigate the damage to brain cell connections). This theory was originally developed by Stern and colleagues and explains how people with less brain reserve capacity and/or with fewer cognitive alternative coping skills could show a faster rate of cognitive decline and faster increased risk of dependence (Stern, 2012). This cognitive reserve (or lack of) has implications for design needs and the opportunities to adapt the home in time to provide optimal support.

Cognitive reserve is associated with education and other early and later life socioeconomic status indicators, such as financial reserve and continued intellectual activities in later life, including reading and using information and communication technology, for instance. These are all protective factors for dementia (Irving et al., 2018). This means that those who need design adaptations most and may develop dementia earlier, also risk not being able to afford these adaptations unless the state, local community or family aids them.

Dementia design as prevention of progression to dependency and to promote mental health

A case could be made that all new built homes should be dementia inclusive, as this would not only benefit mental health in general (e.g. for people living with diagnosed learning disabilities, anxiety, autism or depression), but also benefit the population as a whole, with an abundance of light and calming, simple and open environments that link to green spaces. This proposed part M+ guideline (as a follow-on from part M, for physical disability) was initially proposed by our group.

This could contravene the personalised and creative atmosphere, so homes must also be person-centred, allowing any person who lives there to make cost-effective easy adaptations that suit them safely. Guidelines must be clear, sustainable, energy-efficient and affordable for consumers, but must also be do-able for builders and developers. This is especially important as the costs for building have increased over the last years, with fewer specialist tradesmen to do the jobs required, e.g. experienced joiners, electricians, etc., in the post-Brexit UK.

Design features need to be implemented as preventative factors for progressive decline and dependency, rather than to be done as a crisis response. This was reflected in the comments by stakeholders who visited our Chris and Sally dementia-friendly house in Watford, close to London (Halsall et al., 2023). While middle-aged and younger-old people were much taken with the structural changes of the house (open plan, dementia-inclusive kitchen features, visibility of the bathroom, no thresholds, a lift, etc.), older people (>75) favoured less upheaval and building work, which would also force a temporary moving out. This older group preferred paints and soft furnishings to aid their independence and navigation. Similar results were reported by our Dunhill Medical Trust funded PhD student Barbara Balocating Dunn in a larger multi-ethnic sample across the UK.

So, perhaps all new homes should be 'dementia friendly' or allow easy, cheap, sustainable and energy-efficient adaptations to make them so. This must be done with the occupants the homes are developed for. Better future modelling using artificial intelligence on how fast and severe the progression of functional decline is estimated to be in the individual over time, depending on age, ability, needs preferences, pathological and demographic (reserve) factors, would have important implications for when design changes need to be made to homes, to ensure optimal autonomy and independence across the life course.

While on paper, AD-related changes are, on average, slow and gradual, strokes or other emerging additional pathology (but also stress, such as bereavement or moving to a care home), can accelerate the functional decline and worsen the prognosis unexpectedly and quickly. Being mindful of such issues, by providing support during bereavement and adapting the new home to resemble the original homes' lay-out, including light and furniture placement can perhaps help prevent this catastrophic worsening and decline, that is often seen after such stressors and life events. Anecdotally, where the new home environment was mirrored on the old interior design, and working together with three people living with dementia, the move to the new home did not result in the anticipated worsening of functioning and increased dependency.

Is there benefit of using the traditional medical model vs alternative local methods?

Describing the pathology adds to the recognition of dementia as a medical disease which could be important for stigma reduction, even though it might have limitations in predicting an individual's progression to dependency. In developing rural areas, and in some communities, living with dementia can be seen as the person being possessed, as being childish, obtuse and senile or plain crazy (Porath, 2008). This misunderstanding can lead to abuse, which is much more common in older people living with dementia and their carers than perceived or acknowledged (Weaver, 2018).

Our recent ESRC-funded research showed a wide variety in how older people and their care needs were perceived in Indonesia (Schröder-Butterfill et al., 2023). This ranged from 'successful ageing' or 'deserving a (disempowering) rest' seen in the urban affluent with access to care and support, to invisible frailty and dependency in poor people who often could not afford access to support for their care and medical needs. This can result in complicated situations and dynamics to isolation and neglect of older people without families, to overburdened (usually female) family members needing to provide care with the additional burdens of poverty (Schröder-Butterfill and Fithry, 2014; Schröder-Butterfill et al., 2023). Kaders, community volunteers, are being trained by universities to help provide support and information to carers by Puskesmas (primary health care centres).

Assessment of medical factors driving onset and/or progression of symptoms in individuals

To what extent has the Western medical practice been so very different in their treatment of people living with dementia? Current dementia drugs often only work for a limited period in a small percentage of people, have harmful side-effects (such as brain infections and stroke), are expensive and only work marginally better than placebos. Calming drugs to reduce BPSD and extra care needs in care homes often lead to falls and disorientation, with a worsening of the dementia symptoms (Santiago Martinez et al., 2023).

The main reason for dementia's medicalisation was the hope that we would find a medical treatment to stop the accumulation of pathology leading to functional loss. One of the problems is that Alzheimer's brain pathology builds up in several decades before cognitive and behavioural issues become apparent, by which time it is too late (Jack et al., 2011). Biomarkers used in combination can identify those at risk for developing dementia with a good accuracy (Gunes et al., 2022). However, while combinations of such biomarkers are getting increasingly better at predicting dementia, most still require specialist cerebrospinal fluid extraction, which is not without risk and costs. Again, costly long-term preventative medical treatment and screening would not be accessible to those who might benefit from this most and often live in LMIC rural communities.

In addition, there can be a mismatch between the medical condition (e.g. as reflected by biomarkers) and actual care needs. These care needs can fluctuate, even within the day, but also depend on the care structures and complexities of the environments around the individual, including their needs and habits. When, for instance, we asked people in rural Indonesia in 2005 about dementia, all present stated it did not exist in their villages. When we described individual dementia symptoms, a similar prevalence to that in Western societies was found, of between 5 and 9% in people over 65 years of age (Hogervorst et al., 2011).

The care structures around these rural Indonesian people living with dementia and the low-demand environments (with no technology required for wayfinding, banking, etc.) would suggest that dependency was not regarded as an issue in 2005. Of course, with increasing urban migration of younger people, care needs become an increasing issue for poor, older, rural people, who were also found to be most at risk for dementia and frailty (Hogervorst et al., 2021). In addition, hidden issues of isolation and neglect became apparent when our Indonesian team were invited to visit people's homes, rather than just focus on data from community centres, which only those who had time, the physical ability and money could reach and attend (Schroder-Butterfill et al., 2023).

Similar situations were described by social workers visiting poor older Bangladeshi in Loughborough, who did not attend community centres or

GP because of language and cultural barriers in 2013. To support those who most need it, they must be actively engaged with, but on an equal and respectful level. Shame and/or pride, stigma and/or fierce independence, with both physical and financial inability and technology illiteracy are all barriers to allow positive engagement, which could result in increasingly lower levels of community support and isolation.

Recognising delirium

Dementia is a confusing disease. Often a person living with dementia seems fine in the morning to then, after an exhausting day of impressions, be quite confused with significant cognitive impairments in the afternoon. Some days seem better while others are much worse. It is not always immediately clear what drives change and fluctuation in symptoms.

Changes in behaviour and cognitive functioning can be aggravated by low-level infectious disease, such as urinary tract- or upper respiratory tract infections and are often expressed as a delirium (Bellelli et al., 2021). With one in five older people estimated to not show elevated temperatures, low-grade infections could be missed. This is an important factor, as with antibiotic treatment of bacterial infections, a great deal of cognitive improvement and reduced confusion (delirium) was seen in Oxford Project to Investigate Memory and Ageing participants.

Pain is also associated with delirium, with its fluctuations in cognition, alertness and consciousness, but pain experienced by people with dementia is often not understood by carers, as it is sometimes not communicated verbally by people living with dementia. Other very common issues seen in ageing, such as constipation, low blood pressure (due to continued treatment with anti-hypertensives), heart or kidney failure, insufficient nutrient intake due to issues with teeth and painful dentures, can also lead to delirium These factors need to be diagnosed and treated to maximise cognitive and behavioural ability in the older person, but unfortunately are often not done due to time constraints, lack of medical specialists and the under-recognition of delirium.

A full medical examination should always be carried out, but all too often the diagnosis of dementia (meaning that there are no other medical disorders that better explain the cognitive and behavioural disorders found in the individual) is given without due diligence. In fact, according to most criteria, the dementia diagnosis (other than Lewy body dementia, which comes with fluctuations in alertness and consciousness and confusion with vivid visual hallucinations and cognitive issues) should not be made in the presence of delirium (APA, 1994).

However, delirium is often not recognised, despite being a leading cause of mortality in older people, especially when they present with this in hospitals. With a lack of specialist medical staff in many developing countries, training is now provided to support the recognition of delirium and identify reversible factors that lead to secondary (possible treatable) dementias which include hypofunction of the thyroid, lack of nutrition, etc.

Reliability of the diagnoses of dementia

Even without delirium, we found that dementia diagnostics only had moderate interrater reliability, even between the most experienced neurologists, and moderate validity when live case records were compared to post-mortem confirmed dementias (Hogervorst, 2000). We developed a computerised diagnostic system accounting for all known dementia diagnostic criteria to allow better differential diagnostics and improved reliability and validity of the clinical diagnoses, when compared to the post-mortem confirmed diagnoses (Hogervorst et al., 2003).

While useful for research, clinically this is only useful if targeted treatment would be available or if better modelling of progression could be done to predict when independent living would become difficult. These elements discussed are all indicative of the need for description of a highly personalised dementia journey, but this again reflects the strong socioeconomic divide, as in many countries access to such future predictive modelling of disease progression services would only be available to those who can afford it.

The Chris and Sally home to prevent progression to dependency

Many older people wish to stay home when they age, and this can also be a cost-effective sustainable method of care. The evidence-based Chris and Sally house was a commissioned dementia-inclusive demonstration home based at the BRE in Watford, London and is described in more detail in another book (Halsall et al., 2023). In many ways, this house used the traditional medical model.

For instance, to guide the design of this home, persona were developed to show designers and architects how people living with dementia can have good and bad days, how these fluctuations affect their needs and how their varying and progressive needs can impact on design requirements. We identified the cognitive, sensorimotor and behavioural changes over the different stages of dementia (minimal, mild, moderate to severe) in several steps, together with various service providers and academic specialists. This part of the project was carried out by Charlotte Jais for her PhD, with ergonomics/ health care specialist Prof Sue Hignett and Prof Eef Hogervorst, as dementia expert from Loughborough University.

The house was cost- and energy-efficient and sustainable, with solar panels, shading to prevent glare, insulation and thermal control monitoring systems planned and investigated by civil and building engineers from Loughborough (Prof Malcolm Cook). It was (wheelchair) accessible with open plan living, etc., but also included specific dementia inclusive design by specialist dementia architects, Bill Halsall from Halsall Lloyd Partnership (HLP) and Robert McDonnell from Liverpool John Moores. They used knowledge obtained from their previous projects, which had been guided by people living with dementia, to accommodate and stimulate active and independent living. Manisha Jain funded by the Dunhill Medical Trust and Ahmet Begde funded by the Turkish Research Council investigated whether people living with dementia wanted technology to help with activities of daily life, better memory and psychosocial activities including exercise.

The spaces were calming, with 'dementia specialist' colour schemes from Dulux. While there was little use of the colour red (because the blue-green spectrum colour perception declines, using red in design for orientation was proposed by the Stirling group), it was initially argued that using sufficient light reflective value contrast between features would allow people to navigate the spaces without obstruction, falls and confusion. However, our dementia interior design specialist Janice from HLP countered that splashes of bright colours would have been better to alleviate the dullness that can come with the changes in visual perception with resultant effects on mood.

Patient and Public Involvement and Engagement (PPPIE) input to design and the role of technology

Still, the extra-large windows and interior lights (3x the normal strength) in the Chris and Sally house to improve mood and mitigate the loss of visual contrast sensitivity leading to falls were very well perceived by Patient and Public Involvement and Engagement (PPIE) during inclusive meetings at the home. The spaces created included a downstairs bathroom that could be seen from all angles and also met part M guidelines, which included non-slip, non-threshold, level floors, railings, markings on the stairs, lifts, rounded corners in furniture, glass frontage of cabinets, no clutter, etc. Temperature regulation and optimal indoor environments for people with dementia and their carers were also further investigated by Dunhill Medical Trust sponsored PhD Ahmad Aladawi, Dr Ben Roberts and Prof Malcolm Cook. All people visiting the house at BRE stated they would like to live there. So, good dementia-inclusive design is an all-inclusive design.

Bill Halsall had used co-design by including PPIE to develop and vet the house, from its initial ideas and drawings to 3D models, to the actual demonstration house (Halsall et al., 2023). Together, with the University of Technology in Delft, with Prof Tischa van der Cammen, Dr Armagan Albayrak and Dr Gubing Wang (at the time a PhD student), we also co-created specific features in the house, such as activity chairs. We used cartoons, models, and demonstrations, which led to much improved material, which was then further used in feasibility and acceptability studies.

Personalised designing and care tools

Dr Wang and her colleagues went on to develop the Know-me application which combines materials to apply a personalised dementia inclusive design in a systematic way for designers including a persons' history, family, behaviours, non-pharmacological treatments that work for them, capabilities and other relevant data (Wang et al., 2021). This system can remind designers and architects to collect relevant and personal data. It could also make individual needs visible for care take-over facilitation, much like the sheets of paper hanging behind the beds in the Nightingale care home in India (see Epilogue, this volume). With many staff leaving the profession due to poor pay, little career progression and long working hours, such a quick visual update of needs, red flags and abilities can support the person with dementia and the carer, and allows both to be seen as individuals, rather than the person with dementia being just another case who requires generic care.

The person-centred approach for specialist dementia facility design and care homes

As a significant response to the medical approach and described by Bob Woods in this volume, the person-centred approach, was originally developed by Tom Kitwood (1997). It has seven core values which are individuality, independence, privacy, partnership, choice, dignity, respect and rights. Difficult interactions between patients and care staff are seen as an expression of unmet needs, with difficulty in communicating such needs and receiving appropriate solutions to meet them. This approach was seen to lead to improved quality of life for both carers and people with dementia. Better support and training for care staff using the person-centred approach in hospitals also led to substantial savings including retaining of staff, as Professor Clive Ballard's studies in the UK showed (Halsall et al., 2023).

A true person-centred design approach

Eef Hogervorst met Kevin Charras online during the pandemic (they only met live just before production of this book in October 2024 at the INTERDEM meeting in Helsinki). Kevin's person-centred approach to treat people living with dementia as the person they are, with their own needs and wants, with respect, is incorporated in all his designs. As we have seen, the medical model lacks precision in describing both pathology and clinical progression of individuals. It contrasts with the person-centred approach, which focuses on meeting people's individual needs and wants. This is the theoretical approach used in the subsequent chapters and Charras provides a fuller context for this, describing contemporary streams underlying much of current dementia-inclusive design in his chapter later in Part 1 of this volume.

In-depth box

- The traditional medical model uses distinctions between different types of dementia based on brain pathology and presumed clinical correlates.
- However, the individual journey of people living with dementia needs better modelling to ensure that design flexibly adapts to changes in these needs to promote independence.
- Dementia can fluctuate and express very different between and within people which designers need to be made aware of.
- Delirium needs to be better recognised and treated.
- Personalised approaches in the medical model indicate the need for person-centred adaptation in design.

Acknowledgements

We would like to acknowledge all participants, colleagues and funders of the studies mentioned such as the ESRC, Dunhill Medical Trust, Alzheimer's Research UK, The Turkish Research Council and Loughborough University

References

Alzheimer's Association, 2020. Alzheimer's Disease Facts and Figures. *Alzheimer's & Dementia*, 16 (3), 391–460.

American Psychiatric Association, 1994. *Diagnostic and statistical manual of mental disorders, 4th ed. Diagnostic and statistical manual of mental disorders*, 4th ed. Arlington, VA, US: American Psychiatric Publishing, Inc.

Arifin, E., and Hogervorst, E., 2015. Elderly's Self-Rated Health Status and Functional Capacity at the District Level in Indonesia. *Journal of Population Ageing*. 8. doi:10.1007/s12062-015-9115-1.

Ayodele, T., Rogaeva, E., Kurup, J.T., Beecham, G., and Reitz, C., 2021. Early-onset Alzheimer's disease: What is Missing in Research? *Current Neurology and Neuroscience Reports*, 21 (2), 1–10.

Bellelli, G., Brathwaite, J.S., and Mazzola, P., 2021. Delirium: A Marker of Vulnerability in Older People. *Frontiers in Aging Neuroscience*, 13, 626127.

Emre, M., Aarsland, D., Brown, R., Burn, D.J., Duyckaerts, C., Mizuno, Y., Broe, G.A., Cummings, J., Dickson, D.W., Gauthier, S., Goldman, J., Goetz, C., Korczyn, A., Lees, A., Levy, R., Litvan, I., McKeith, I., Olanow, W., Poewe, W., Quinn, N., Sampaio, C., Tolosa, E., and Dubois, B., 2007. Clinical Diagnostic Criteria for Dementia Associated with Parkinson's Disease. *Movement Disorders: Official Journal of the Movement Disorder Society*, 22 (12), 1689–1707.

Gunes, S., Aizawa, Y., Sugashi, T., Sugimoto, M., and Rodrigues, P.P., 2022. Biomarkers for Alzheimer's Disease in the Current State: A Narrative Review. *International Journal of Molecular Sciences*, 23 (9), Art. No.: 4962.

Halsall, B., Riley, M., and Hogervorst, E., 2023. *Design for Dementia: Living Well at Home*. Routledge: London

Hippius, H. and Neundörfer, G., 2003. The Discovery of Alzheimer's Disease. *Dialogues in Clinical Neuroscience*, 5 (1), 101–108.

Hogervorst, E., Bandelow, S., Combrinck, M., Irani, S., and Smith, A.D., 2003. The Validity and Reliability of 6 Sets of Clinical Criteria to Classify Alzheimer's Disease and Vascular Dementia in Cases Confirmed Post-mortem: Added Value of a Decision Tree Approach. *Dementia and Geriatric Cognitive Disorders*, 16 (3), 170–180.

Hogervorst, E., Barnetson, L., Jobst, K.A., Nagy, Z., Combrinck, M., and Smith, A.D., 2000. Diagnosing Dementia: Interrater Reliability Assessment and Accuracy of the NINCDS/ADRDA Criteria versus CERAD Histopathological Criteria for Alzheimer's Disease. *Dementia and Geriatric Cognitive Disorders*, 11 (2), 107–113.

Hogervorst, E., Mursjid, F., Ismail, R.I., Prasetyo, S., Nasrun, M., Mochtar, Ninuk, T., Bandelow, S., Subarkah, Kusdhany, L., and Rahardjo, T.B.W., 2011. Validation of Two Short Dementia Screening Tests in Indonesia. In: S. Jacobsen, ed. *Vascular Dementia: Risk factors, Diagnosis and Treatment*. New York: Nova Science, 235–256.

Hogervorst, E., Schröder-Butterfill, E., Handajani, Y., Kreager, P., and Rahardjo, TB., 2021. Dementia and Dependency vs. Proxy Indicators of the Active Ageing Index in Indonesia. *International Journal of Environmental Research and Public Health*, 18 (16), 8235. doi:10.3390/ijerph18168235.

Irving, K., Hogervorst, E., Oliveira, D., Kivipelto, M, eds., 2018. *New Developments in Dementia Prevention Research: State of the Art and Future Possibilities*. London: Routledge.

Jack, C.R., Albert, M.S., Knopman, D.S., McKhann, G.M., Sperling, R.A., Carrillo, M.C., Thies, B., and Phelps, C.H., 2011. Introduction to the Recommendations from the National Institute on Aging-Alzheimer's Association Workgroups on Diagnostic Guidelines for Alzheimer's Disease. *Alzheimer's & Dementia*, 7 (3), 257–262.

Jain, M. and Hogervorst, E., n.d. Diagnostic and Prevalence Estimates of Dementia in Indonesia: Commentary on "Comprehensive Measurement of the Prevalence of Dementia in Low- and Middle-income Countries: STRiDE Methodology and its Application in Indonesia and South Africa" (In preparation).

Kitwood, T., 1997. *Dementia Reconsidered: The Person Comes First*. Buckingham: Open University Press.

Livingston, G., Huntley, J., Sommerlad, A., Ames, D., Ballard, C., Banerjee, S., Brayne, C., Burns, A., Cohen-Mansfield, J., Cooper, C., Costafreda, S.G., Dias, A., Fox, N., Gitlin, L.N., Howard, R., Kales, H.C., Kivimäki, M., Larson, E.B., Ogunniyi, A., Orgeta, V., Ritchie, K., Rockwood, K., Sampson, E.L., Samus, Q., Schneider, L.S., Selbæk, G., Teri, L., and Mukadam, N., 2020. Dementia Prevention, Intervention, and Care: 2020 Report of the Lancet Commission. *The Lancet*, 396 (10248), 413–446.

McKeith, I. G., Boeve, B. F., Dickson, D. W., Halliday, G., Taylor, J. P., Weintraub, D., Aarsland, D., Galvin, J., Attems, J., Ballard, C. G., Bayston, A., Beach, T. G., Blanc, F., Bohnen, N., Bonanni, L., Bras, J., Brundin, P., Burn, D., Chen-Plotkin, A., Duda, J. E., El-Agnaf, O., Feldman, H., Ferman, T.J., Ffytche, D., Fujishiro, H., Galasko, D., Goldman, J.G., Gomperts, S.N., Graff-Radford, N.R., Honig, L.S., Iranzo, A., Kantarci, K., Kaufer, D., Kukull, W., Lee, V.M.Y., Leverenz, J.B., Lewis, S., Lippa, C., Lunde, A., Masellis, M., Masliah, E., McLean, P., Mollenhauer, B., Montine, T.J., Moreno, E., Mori, E., Murray, M., O'Brien, J.T., Orimo, S., Postuma, R.B., Ramaswamy, S., Ross, O.A., Salmon, D.P., Singleton, A., Taylor, A., Thomas, A., Tiraboschi, P., Toledo, J.B., Trojanowski, J.Q., Tsuang, D. Walker, Z.,

Yamada, M., and Kosaka, K., 2017. Diagnosis and Management of Dementia with Lewy Bodies: Fourth Consensus Report of the DLB Consortium. *Neurology*, 89 (1), 88–100. doi:10.1212/WNL.0000000000004058.

McKeith, I.G., Galasko, D., Kosaka, K., Perry, E.K., Dickson, D.W., Hansen, L.A., Salmon, D.P., Lowe, J., Mirra, S.S., Byrne, E.J., Lennox, G., Quinn, N.P., Edwardson, J.A., Ince, P.G., Bergeron, C., Burns, A., Miller, B.L., Lovestone, S., Collerton, D., Jansen, E.N.H., Ballard, C., De Vos, R.A.I., Wilcock, G.K., Jellinger, K.A., and Perry, R.H., 1996. Consensus Guidelines for the Clinical and Pathologic Diagnosis of Dementia with Lewy Bodies (DLB): Report of the Consortium on DLB International Workshop. *Neurology*, 47 (5), 1113–1124.

McKhann, G., Drachman, D., Folstein, M., Katzman, R., Price, D., and Stadlan, E.M., 1984. Clinical Diagnosis of Alzheimer's Disease: Report of the NINCDS-ADRDA Work Group* under the Auspices of Department of Health and Human Services Task Force on Alzheimer's Disease. *Neurology*, 34 (7), 939–944.

Menšíková, K., Matěj, R., Colosimo, C., Rosales, R., Tučková, L., Ehrmann, J., Hraboš, D., Kolaříková, K., Vodička, R., Vrtěl, R., Procházka, M., Nevrlý, M., Kaiserová, M., Kurčová, S., Otruba, P., and Kaňovský, P., 2022. Lewy Body Disease or Diseases with Lewy Bodies? *NPJ Parkinsons Dis*ease, 8, 3. doi:10.1038/s41531-021-00273-9.

National Institute on Aging, 2021. *What is Lewy Body Dementia? Causes, Symptoms, and Treatments* [online]. Available from: https://www.nia.nih.gov/health/lewy-body-dementia/what-lewy-body-dementia-causes-symptoms-and-treatments [Accessed 13 Jan 2024].

Porath, N., 2008. The Naturalization of Psychiatry in Indonesia and its Interaction with Indigenous Therapeutics. *Bijdragen tot de Taal-, Land- en Volkenkunde*, 164 (4), 500–528.

Santiago Martinez, P., Lord, S.R., Close, J.C.T., and Taylor, M.E., 2023. Associations between Psychotropic and Anti-dementia Medication Use and Falls in Community-dwelling Older Adults with Cognitive Impairment. *Archives of Gerontology and Geriatrics*, 114.

Schröder-Butterfill, E. and Fithry, T.S., 2014. Care Dependence in Old Age: Preferences, Practices and Implications in Two Indonesian Communities. *Ageing and Society*, 34 (3), 361.

Schröder-Butterfill, E., Porath, N., Handajani, Y.S., Larastiti, C., Delpada, B., Hogervorst, E., Insriani, H., Jelly, Kreager, P., Rahayuningtyas, D., Sare, Y., and Tresno., 2023. Vulnerable, Heroic … or Invisible? Representations versus Realities of Later Life in Indonesia. *Progress in Development Studies*, 23 (4), 408–426. doi:10.1177/14649934231197277.

Stern, Y., 2012. Cognitive Reserve in Ageing and Alzheimer's Disease. *The Lancet. Neurology*, 11 (11), 1006–1012.

Wang, G., Albayrak, A., Hogervorst, E., and van der Cammen, T. J. M., 2021. Know-Me: A Toolkit for Designing Personalised Dementia Care. *International Journal of Environmental Research and Public Health*, 18 (11), 5662. https://doi.org/10.3390/ijerph18115662.

Wang, X., Bakulski, K.M., Paulson, H.L., Albin, R.L., and Park, S.K., 2023. Associations of Healthy Lifestyle and Socioeconomic Status with Cognitive

Function in U.S. Older Adults. *medRxiv: The Preprint Server for Health Sciences*, 2023.01.24.23284961. doi:10.1101/2023.01.24.23284961.

Weaver, D., 2018. Dementia's Hidden Darkness: Violence and Domestic Abuse [online]. Available from: https://theconversation.com/dementias-hidden-darkness-violence-and-domestic-abuse-104308 [Accessed 13 Jan 2024].

Wiederkehr, S., Simard, M., Fortin, C., and Van Reekum, R., 2008. Validity of the Clinical Diagnostic Criteria for Vascular Dementia: A Critical Review. Part II. *Journal of Neuropsychiatry and Clinical Neurosciences*, 20 (2), 162–177.

Wingo, T.S., Lah, J.J., Levey, A.I., and Cutler, D.J., 2012. Autosomal Recessive Causes Likely in Early-Onset Alzheimer Disease. *Archives of Neurology*, 69 (1), 59–64.

2

Creating homes for individuals living with dementia

The past, the present and the future

Margaret Calkins

Introduction

The approach and values guiding the design of shared residential or long-term care environments for people living with dementia has undergone several major transitional periods over the past 50 years. The early designs of these settings did not occur in a vacuum. There were numerous pressures, from the movement to close mental hospitals to the growing recognition that people living with dementia often did not fit the profile of residents of nursing homes who needed primarily clinical care and support, which spurred innovation in design. There were also publications, a few articles at first in the 1970s and 1980s, then several books, which set forth values and principles for designing for these individuals. As more projects were built, several books analyzed early care settings designed specifically for people living with dementia through the lens of these principles. The focus of this chapter is on the development of dementia-specific nursing and care homes in the North America, Northern Europe, and Australia, the values and principles that guide their design, and how this has changed over time.

In the 1950s through 1970s, nursing homes and other care homes (hereafter referred to as nursing/care homes) did not generally segregate out different sub-groups of residents based on diagnosis or condition, and buildings were designed to reflect a medical model of care (Calkins et al., 2024; Judd et al., 1998). Subsequently, based in part on the work of M. Powell Lawton in the early 1970s, it was increasingly thought that the care needs of these individuals were significantly different from those of traditional residents of long-term care, whose needs were primarily for physical care. This spurred the development of what was generally referred to as "Special Care Units" (SCUs) in the US, and by various names in other countries. While this practice of segregating people living with dementia from people who are experiencing primarily physical/medical challenges continues, there has also been a significant shift in the underlying assumption that the needs of people living with dementia are substantially different from the needs of people currently not experiencing the symptoms of dementia. In the US, this shift in thinking began in

DOI: 10.4324/9781003416241-4

earnest in the 1990s, variously being called culture change, person-centered care, resident-directed care, and self-directed, relationship-based living. As this philosophy of care becomes more widely adopted, innovation in the design of care settings continues. This chapter explores these shifts in values and practices which inform the creation of nursing/care homes for people living with dementia in Northern Europe, Australia, and the US.

Theoretical background

The earliest work in this area was by M. Powell Lawton, both with the development of the Environmental Docility Hypothesis (also known as the Competence-Press Model) and the design and subsequent evaluation of the Weiss Pavilion at the Philadelphia Geriatric Center, both in the 1970s (Lawton & Nahemow, 1973; Liebowitz et al., 1979a, 1979b). The Competence-Press Model is one of the most widely cited models exploring the interwoven relationship between older individuals and their environment. It posits that individuals have certain levels of competencies that enable them to respond either effectively or ineffectively to environmental demands (press). Competencies are multi-faceted and variable and include biological health, sensorimotor functioning, cognitive skills, and ego strength. Similarly, environmental press is comprised of multiple elements, though these are not well defined by Lawton & Nahemow (1973). In basic terms, there is a theoretical mean adaptation line, where the abilities of the individual are in equilibrium with the press of the environment- a place of homeostasis. Modest changes in press, either higher or lower, are still within a zone of positive affect and adaptive behavior. However, when the environmental press is either significantly too high (overstimulating) or too low (sensory deprivation), the individual experiences negative affect and maladaptive behavior. An individual with high competencies has wide latitude in coping with greater amounts environmental press while staying within the comfort zone of positive affect and adaptive behavior. As competencies decrease, however, the overall amount of press that can be managed decreases as does the effective range of press that allows a person to remain in the zone of positive affect and adaptive behavior.

This model has been widely applied in the consideration of settings for people living with dementia, who are generally considered in the lower-competent range. The model posits they are much more sensitive to too much stimulation, especially stimulation that is challenging for them to understand. This was often translated to mean that a very low stimulus environment would be appropriate. However, one of the limitations of this model is that it doesn't easily address the reality that each individual has different levels of competencies in interdependent areas of functioning (physical vs. cognitive, for instance). Many individuals living with dementia in nursing/care homes are quite functional on a physical level, able to walk long distances with ease. Similarly, the model tends to conceptualize "press" in terms of amount, but not form. Carp (1976) suggested that the environment needs to be seen not only in terms of press or amount of stimulation, but also as a resource that can be used prosthetically to compensate for deficits.

Much of the thinking from this model was used in the design of the Weiss Pavilion at the Philadelphia Geriatric Center. Recognizing that wayfinding skills are a common symptom of many forms of dementia, the traditional long double-loaded corridor was eliminated in favor of an open plan with bedrooms arranged about a 40 × 100 (12m × 30m) space, with social spaces and the nursing station being highly visible from all areas (Lawton, 1986; Liebowitz et al., 1979b). The evaluation of the setting, while constrained by many factors, did suggest the environment had a prosthetic effect, as several behavioral indicators, such as engagement in enriching activities, greater angle of gaze (looking around) and less "pathological" behavior were found, while the cognitive trajectory of residents continued to decline (Lawton, 1986; Liebowitz et al., 1979b). The most significant take-away of this experimental setting was the evidence that the traditional medical model of design of nursing/care homes might not be supportive of the needs and abilities of individuals living with dementia and that other approaches needed to be explored.

Early influential publications

The first book on designing for people living with dementia was published in 1988 (see more, below), but there had been a number of printed resources written prior to that. In the US, beyond the influential early work of Lawton, Mace and Rabins authored the highly influential *36 Hour Day* (Mace & Rabins, 1981), though it mostly focused on care issues, with only a short section on shared residential environments. Hiatt, Coons, and others authored a number of publications on long-term care design, several of which were specifically focused on settings for people living with dementia (Calkins, 1987; Coons, 1988; Coons & Weaverdyck, 1986; Gutman, 1989; Hiatt-Snyder et al., 1978; L. Hiatt, 1985; L. G. Hiatt, 1980; Schultz, 1987). In Australia, a Department of Health New South Wales Report, published in 1983 (Richmond, 1983) as the country sought to close mental hospitals, provided the basic framework for multidisciplinary care in "human scale" facilities (Fleming & Bowles, 1987). There were also publications around the design and evaluation of C.A.D.E. (Confused and Disturbed Elderly) units (Fleming & Bowles, 1987; Fleming et al., 1989). Fewer publications from the 1980s were identified from Northern Europe (Benjamin & Spector, 1990; Keen, 1989; Pritchard, 1990). In England, the *Journal of Dementia Care*, which regularly featured articles that addressed various design issues didn't start publishing until 1993.

The first comprehensive examination of design principles was *Design for Dementia: Planning Environments for the Elderly and Confused* published in

1988 (Calkins, 1988). It argued that care settings need to be conceptualized holistically, with a tri-partite model that includes the people in the setting (individuals living with dementia, their care partners and others), the organization (policies, procedures, and culture), and the physical/designed environment (components such as walls and furnishings, and sensory and spatial properties, such as lighting and sounds). The book then identified five "Environment and Behavior" issues which formed the basis for a series of specific recommendations. Several building examples were used to illustrate features; however, this was sufficiently early in the evolution of the field that there were very few extant examples available, especially examples of complete buildings (vs. relatively minor modifications made to traditional nursing/care homes). The first two environmental intervention strategies identified were to create a homelike environment and provide prosthetic supports to compensate for impaired functioning.

Written resources on the design of care settings for people living with dementia burgeoned in the 1990s and are too numerous to list out. However, there were three pivotal books that further laid out foundational values for designing for dementia, values which have remained very consistent over the subsequent 35 years. In 1991, Cohen and Weisman's landmark book *Holding on to Home* was published (Cohen & Weisman, 1991), which defined four "General Attributes" of the environment: non-institutional character, eliminating environmental barriers, things from the past, and sensory stimulation without stress. These were then expounded upon when examining overall building organization and specific activity areas/rooms in a nursing/care setting, which addressed more subtle goals such as "opportunities for meaningful wandering" and public to private realms. Cohen and Weisman explored a broader continuum of settings, from homes in the community to day and respite programs, group homes, and free-standing care centers. They included seven prototypical designs, which demonstrated how the different broad attributes and smaller goals can be integrated to make manifest the "relationship between basic concepts, rooted in therapeutic and organizational goals, and resultant architectural form" (Cohen & Weisman, 1991, p. 129). A companion book was published two years later, *Contemporary Environments for People with Dementia* (Cohen & Day, 1993), which applied the principles from *Holding on to Home* to 11 care settings and one garden, primarily from the US, with one from Australia and one from Canada. The majority of projects had been built between 1987 and 1993, demonstrating the significant growth in the field between the publication of *Design for Dementia* in 1988 and 1993.

The fourth influential book, also titled *Design for Dementia* was a collaboration between three Australian and UK experts (Judd et al., 1998), and is similar to Cohen and Day (1993) in that it is an analysis of 20 dementia care communities from Northern Europe and Australia. Coming several years after the previous publications, there were significantly more projects available to review. Projects were selected because they generally fit the authors' shared set of values, though interestingly, at the front of the book each author presents their own set of values and design strategies, which have some consistency but are clearly conceptualized and structured in different ways. Unfortunately, they do not give dates of when these care homes were built or opened, so it is more difficult to estimate when the shift away from more traditional medical models began.

Design principles

Clearly, there was growing international support that the medical model wasn't the only, and likely not the best, model particularly for persons living with dementia. There is a bit of a chicken and egg issue, which came first: clearly articulated design principles, or innovative designs? The answer is probably a bit of both. This section will address primarily the values as they were articulated in the four books mentioned above, followed in the next section by a description of how these values were applied.

Despite being developed on different continents, there are more similarities than disparities between the values articulated by these early book authors (see Table 2.1). Each author used their own phrases, and they reflect a mix of person-centered goals (e.g., orientation) and design strategies (e.g., cues). Every author started with reducing the scale and creating a domestic/homelike ambiance as the top priority. This is likely both a response to the highly clinical/institutional elements that characterize the other alternatives available at the time, and a deep recognition that an environment that reflects home will provide more familiar resources so individuals living with dementia can draw upon long-term memory to make sense of their setting. This is now referred to, generally, as a household model (vs. medical or institutional). Orientation, wayfinding, and provision of cues were also mentioned by all five authors, in recognition that disorientation is a hallmark symptom that can cause significant distress but is also highly impacted by environment elements such as overall layout with visible destinations, décor that clearly identifies the purpose of different spaces, and the presences of cues and signage. Cohen and Weisman refer to this value as opportunities for meaningful wandering, arguing that much of what is termed "wandering" is a result of an illegible environment and thus improving legibility will reduce this behavioral response. There is also agreement amongst most of the authors on the importance of designing so the environment supports functional activities instead of becoming a barrier. Similarly, designing to support personalization, enabling residents to live with their own possessions as a reflection of who they are, as a person, is mentioned in all four books. The presence, accessibility, and design of outdoor spaces which offer both opportunities for autonomy (deciding whether to be inside or outside) and positive engagement (gardening, birdwatching, etc.) was mentioned by all authors but one.

Table 2.1 Design principles from pivotal early books

Calkins, 1988	Cohen & Weisman, 1991	Cohen & Day 1993	Judd et al., 1998		
			Marshall	Judd	Phippen
Environment & behavior issues	General attributes of the environment	General attributes of the environment	Principles	Objectives	
Homelike environment	Non-institutional character	Noninstitutional image	Small size	Environment should be small	Domestic character (siting, entrances, shared spaces, kitchen, dining arrangements, personal space)
	Clusters of small activity spaces	family clusters	Familiar, domestic		
	Public to private realms	Public to private realms		Environment should be familiar	
Wayfinding/ Orientation	Opportunities for meaningful wandering	Opportunities for meaningful wandering	Orienting and understandable	Environment should be legible	Cueing
Competence in daily activities	Eliminating environmental barriers	More negotiable environments	Maximize independence	Promote Improvement	
(addresses design strategies of outdoor spaces)	Positive outdoor spaces	Positive outdoor spaces	Safe outdoor space		Design of outside spaces
Personalization	Things from the past	Things from the past	Reinforce personal identify		
			Single rooms with space for personalization		

(Continued)

Table 2.1 (Continued)

Calkins, 1988	Cohen & Weisman, 1991	Cohen & Day 1993	Judd et al., 1998		
			Marshall	Judd	Phippen
Environment & behavior issues	General attributes of the environment	General attributes of the environment	Principles	Objectives	
Respite areas	Staff retreat	Retreat for staff members	Care for staff		
Privacy/ socialization	Clusters of small activity spaces	Places for visiting			
Safety/security			Unobtrusive concerns for safety	Environment must be safe	
Prosthetic Support			Compensate for disability	Compensate for individual dysfunction	
	Sensory stimulation without stress	Sensory stimulation without stress	Controlled stimuli-particularly noise.		
			Enhance self-esteem and confidence	Environment should promote self-esteem, autonomy and individuality	
	Other living things (plants and pets)		Welcome relatives and local communities		

Finally, all four books also recognize that staff are an integral part of the setting, and the environment needs to both support this work, and provide a place of respite from the rigors of the work. The remaining design principles, privacy and socialization, control of excess stimulation, support for autonomy and self-confidence, and connection to other living things (people, pets and plants) are mentioned in one or two of the books. A discussion was held in the spring of 2023 with eight individuals living with dementia, some still at home and some in shared residential settings, to review what their priorities are in the design of shared residential settings. Residential scale/looking like a house with private bedrooms were at the top of the list, along with being able to go outside when they wanted (not just when it was convenient for staff), and not being or feeling locked in.

Application of the principles to early design projects

Contemporaneous with the development of the principles, progressive care communities were building, and sometimes evaluating, settings for people living with dementia. The Weiss Pavilion, described above, which opened in 1972 was likely the earliest such setting. While it was revolutionary at the time, it primarily still reflected many aspects of a traditional medical model: it accommodated 40 residents, primarily in double-occupancy bedrooms, and did not convey a residential style of design. Friendship House of Cedar Lake Home, which opened in 1976, was likely the first purpose-built dementia nursing/care home that radically reduced the scale of the setting, accommodating 16 residents in each wing, though the rest of the design reflected the traditional medical model design elements. While a number of dementia-care programs opened in the US in the 1980s, the vast majority were converted wings of existing nursing homes and did not deeply reflect the design principles described above. Two projects opened in 1988 and 1991, the Corinne Dolan Center and Woodside Place, were the first to really apply the principles in the household model of domestic scale (12 and 10 residents in each group, respectively), residential design (fully functional kitchens from which at least some of the meals were prepared, living and dining rooms and private bedrooms) (Calkins, 1993; Cohen & Day, 1993). The other projects in the US described by Cohen and Day did not closely adhere to many of the principles described above: they tended to accommodate more than 20 residents, often did not have residential style kitchens that prepared meals or invited residents' participation and often had shared bedrooms and medical model style and finishes.

In Australia, there were several pioneers, including Richard Fleming, Brian Moss, and Brian Kidd, who developed a number of dementia-specific care homes that differed from the traditional model. The first C.A.D.E (Confused And Disturbed Elderly) unit opened in 1987 and is described as "small units built to provide as near a homelike environment as can be achieved within the restraints imposed by economies of scale and the principles used to reduce confusion" (Fleming & Bowles, 1987, p. 26). Each C.A.D.E. unit accommodated eight residents (though often two were placed back-to-back to allow for staffing efficiencies at night) and had residential spaces (kitchen, dining, lounges, laundry, private bedrooms). C.A.D.E. units were also intended to be located in the middle of communities, so residents could continue to participate in everyday life. In an evaluation of an early C.A.D.E. home, residents showed significant improvement on the Psychogeriatric Rating Scale over a period of 15 months (Fleming et al., 1989). The book by Judd and colleagues describes eight other projects built before 1998. While projects were obviously selected because they reflected the authors' values, it is striking to note that the largest grouping of residents was 14, with most accommodating 8–10 residents, one as few as six. All reflected a household model and had between two and five living areas (groupings of residents) that were adjacent or, more typically, connected.

In Northern Europe, Judd and colleagues similarly identify 12 projects that all reflect many elements of household models, with living areas that generally accommodate six to eight residents, with a few as high as 10, private bedrooms, functional and accessible kitchens, and residential décor (Judd et al., 1998). Most are well situated in existing neighborhoods, providing both a familiar context and often opportunities to do local shopping or community activities. Only one project accommodated 13 residents in a single group and provided an equal number of private and shared bedrooms.

Current principles and designs

Since the late 1980s when the movement toward specialized care settings for people living with dementia started gaining traction, there are some elements that show substantial changes, and some aspects that have remained largely consistent. The basic principles laid out in the four pivotal books described earlier are largely intact, though our language and thinking have evolved in many ways (we don't refer to them as the demented or "confused and disturbed elderly"). Much of the focus then was on "deinstitutionalizing" the setting and managing behaviors and symptoms of dementia such as wandering and safety concerns. Today the focus is much more on the well-being of residents and their care partners (both staff and families) by supporting continued engagement in meaningful relationships and pursuits. A review of currently promulgated design guides for dementia care settings, from a variety of sources including Alzheimer's Associations/Societies, university/academic centers, and government-sponsored web-based resources show that there continues to be a focus on creating settings that reflect home and compensate for changes that accompany people's journey through dementia (Calkins, 2018; Dementia Australia, 2022; Fisher et al., 2022; Gan et al., 2021; Halsall & MacDonald, 2017; Schmachtenberg et al., 2022).

A particularly well-articulated set of design principles is available in the World Alzheimer Report 2020 (Zeisel et al., 2020), which takes a comprehensive look at the history, trajectories, and current status of designing for individuals living with dementia. It is worth noting that their design principles came from early work by Fleming in 1987 (Fleming & Bowles, 1987), which have been further developed and expanded upon in the intervening years. Their principles include the following: unobtrusively reduce risks; provide a human scale; allow people to see and be seen; reduce unhelpful stimulation; optimize helpful stimulation; support movement and engagement; create a familiar place; provide opportunities to be alone or with others; link to community; design in response to vision for way of life. Comparing this with the principles in Table 2.1, only "allow people to see and be seen" and "Design in response to vision for way of life" are new additions.

The language has evolved and shifted to reflect a greater respect for the dignity and personhood of each individual. Some concepts are given more consideration, for example, risk-taking. In the 1980s and 1990s, while autonomy and the opportunity to make decisions were included, there was a more prevailing attitude that people living with dementia needed to be protected from making bad or risky decisions. Today, there is greater recognition that people have the right to take risks. Ensuring they understand both the upside benefit and the downside risk of a decision is part of good care, but in the end, the individual has the right to self-determination, as long as it doesn't put others at risk. Similarly, there is a greater emphasis today on inclusion of people living with dementia in everything that touches their lives: "Nothing about me without me" is the tag line for Dementia Alliance International (DAI, 2021), one of several organizations developed and operated _by_ people living with dementia, _for_ people living with dementia. The scope of settings that are considered part of this field has also expanded: community accessibility/livability is also receiving greater focus, with age-friendly and dementia-friendly initiatives occurring world-wide (Darlington et al., 2021; Gordon et al., 2016; Pozo Menéndez & Higueras García, 2022; Wu et al., 2019).

In terms of actual designs, there is both a continuation of the approaches illustrated in the two-design review books mentioned above and a few more radical innovations. While there are numerous publications that showcase a few dementia-specific designs, the most comprehensive recent publication is the World Alzheimer Report 2020 (Zeisel et al., 2020), which provides case studies of 61 residential care settings, in addition to a smaller number of hospitals and public buildings (which are not addressed here) in 27 different countries. Similar to the two books published in the 1990s and described above, each project is described, with floor plans, photos, and a summary of which principles were most influential in the design. It provides a very useful description of settings for people living with dementia, from the 1980s to present day.

Small size and domestic character to the interior design (which includes a functional kitchen) continue to be prominently featured, although there are a number of projects in the World Alzheimer Report 2020 where the number of residents sharing a living area is larger in scale than what the principles generally suggest: 14 is not uncommon, and several are even larger. A number of projects still feature side-by-side shared bedrooms, which offer little privacy or control over personal territory and are contrary to the principles in Table 2.1. It is worth noting that, particularly in the US and Canada, the household model is still viewed with skepticism by many care providers, who continue to cling to traditional medical model buildings, albeit sometimes dressed up with prettier decors. The Green House Project™ is likely the most well-known and fully developed household model. The first Green House home opened in 2003 in Tupelo Mississippi, and yet there are only around 375 Green House homes in operation in 2023. There are other similar projects which chose not to affiliate with the Green House Project, but together these probably comprise less than 10% of all nursing/care homes in the US.

Another area that shows modest innovations relates to outdoor spaces. Access to the outdoors continues to be very important, and creative designs that offer both active and passive engagement are more common. There are now a number of care communities where each resident bedroom has a door that leads directly to outdoor space, providing significantly more autonomy and self-determination (risk-taking) than was evident in the past.

There are also some deeper innovations. Green Care Farms are gaining in popularity, both in the literature (over 1100 references found in an online search) and in operational care settings. They operate either as day programs or as 24-hour programs for extended periods of time. In the Netherlands, Norway, and France, there are over 1,000 green care farms offering day programs, and a smaller number of residential green care farms (Nowak et al., 2015). The residents engage with all farm-related activities and chores such as planting, gardening and harvesting, cooking and canning, and caring for animals (including livestock) and the property. Green Care Farms appear to be most common in Northern Europe, but are also in North America, Asia, and other locations.

The other more radical design innovation is the development of dementia villages. In addition to the spaces one would typically find in a home, there are venues for community spaces, such as cafes/pubs, shops for grocery and pharmacy, a hairdresser, library, possibly health care clinic, sports/gym space for working out, and restaurant. The first such project, De Hogeweyk (also referred to as Hogewey Dementia Village) in The Netherlands, opened in 2008. The village accommodates between 150 and 249 residents, in 23 households of 6–7 residents, each with two bathrooms and a kitchen and has more than 30 clubs that people can join. Residents are free to go anywhere in the village they want, at any time, as there is an unobtrusive secure perimeter. There are now similar dementia villages in several northern European countries, Canada and the US. The goal is to support people to continue to live the life they want to live, regardless of, or perhaps because of the fact that they are living with dementia.

Conclusion

French journalist and writer Jean-Baptiste Alphonse Karr wrote in the January 1849 issue of Les Guêpes (The Wasps) "plus ça change, plus c'est la même chose " – the more things change, the more they stay the same. The previous section ended with a discussion of what would seem to be two very different and innovative types of care settings. And yet, they are really just an extension of the values and principles that were first laid out in the 1980s and early 1990s. It can be argued that there were two significant early changes. The first (which came even before there were settings specifically designed for individuals living with dementias) was recognizing that the settings that had been designed for decades, what is typically referred to as institutional or medical model designs, are fundamentally antithetical to long-stay environments for people living with dementia. The second, and related change, was recognizing that people living with dementia are people first and want the same things that people who are not living with dementia want: to be respected, to have autonomy to make decisions, both major life decisions and everyday decisions about when to wake up or what to have for breakfast, to have options of where to spend time and do things they enjoy doing. They do not need "special" care settings, as they were called in the US. They need what we all need, with a few extra supports to compensate for cognitive changes that occur with progressive neurodegenerative conditions.

It is not the purpose of this chapter to demonstrate the efficacy of these designs, but there is substantial evidence from numerous research projects and scoping reviews that small-scale homelike settings, often referred to as household models, are associated with more positive resident and staff well-being outcomes, at least comparable clinical outcomes, and can be operated for no more money than traditional medical model settings (Bourdon et al., 2022; Chaudhury et al., 2017; Krier et al., 2023; Marquardt et al., 2014). The challenge facing designers, providers, and policymakers now is how to best manage the elimination of the old institutional building stock and move to small household-based designs.

In-depth box

- Met with eight individuals from Dementia Minds group to discuss what is important to them in the design of a shared residential care setting. Their values were aligned with the design principles presented in chapter.
- Includes insights from 35 years of visiting dementia care settings in the US and abroad.

References

Benjamin, L. C., & Spector, J. (1990). Environments for the dementing. *International Journal of Geriatric Psychiatry, 5*, 15–24.

Bourdon, E., Havreng-Théry, C., Lafuente, C., & Belmin, J. (2022, November 1). Effect of the physical environment on health and well-being of nursing homes residents: A scoping review. *Journal of the American Medical Directors Association, 23*(11), 1826.e1821–1826.e1820. https://doi.org/https://doi.org/10.1016/j.jamda.2022.05.026

Calkins, M., Kaup, M., & Abushousheh, A. (2024). Aging and place in the context of shared senior residential settings In M. C. G. Rowles (Ed.), *Handbook of aging and place*. Edward Elgar Publishing Ltd.

Calkins, M. P. (1987). Designing special care units: A systemic approach. *The American Journal of Alzheimer's Care and Research, 2*(2 and 3), 16–22, 30–34.

Calkins, M. P. (1988). *Design for dementia: Planning environments for the elderly and the confused*. National Health Publishing.

Calkins, M. P. (1993). Collaboration in research and design: The Corinne Dolan Alzheimer Center. *Design Research News, XXIV*(1), 8–9.

Calkins, M. P. (2018). From research to application: Supportive and therapeutic environments for people living with dementia. *The Gerontologist, 58*(Supplement 1), S114–S128. https://doi.org/10.1093/geront/gnx146

Carp, F. M. (1976). Housing and living environments of older people. *Handbook of Aging and the Social Sciences, 2*, 44–71.

Chaudhury, H., Cooke, H., Cowie, H., & Razaghi, L. (2017, Advance Access publication March 10, 2017). The influence of the physical environment on residents with dementia in long-term care settings: A review of the empirical literature. *The Gerontologist, 58*(5), e325–e337. https://doi.org/https://doi.org/10.1093/geront/gnw259

Cohen, U., & Day, K. (1993). *Contemporary environments for people with dementia*. Johns Hopkins University Press.

Cohen, U., & Weisman, J. (1991). *Holding on to home: Designing environments for people with dementia*. Johns Hopkins University Press.

Coons, D. (1988). Wandering. *The American Journal of Alzheimer's Care & Related Disorders and Research, 3*(1), 31–36.

Coons, D., & Weaverdyck, S. (1986). Wesley Hall: A residential unit for persons with Alzheimer's disease and related disorders. *Physical and Occupational Therapy in Geriatrics, 4*(3), 29–53.

DAI. (2021). *Dementia alliance international*. Retrieved February 5, 2024, from https://dementiaallianceinternational.org/

Darlington, N., Arthur, A., Woodward, M., Buckner, S., Killett, A., Lafortune, L., Mathie, E., Mayrhofer, A., Thurman, J., & Goodman, C. (2021). A survey of the experience of living with dementia in a dementia-friendly community. *Dementia, 20*(5), 1711–1722.

Dementia Australia. (2022). *Designing for people with dementia*. Department of Health, Victoria, AU Retrieved May 18, 2023, from https://www.health.vic.gov.au/

dementia-friendly-environments/designing-for-people-with-dementia#designing-for-people-with-dementia

Fisher, T., Garley, C., & Morgan, N. (2022). *Dementia and co-creation*. A. s. Society. https://www.alzheimers.org.uk/research/our-research/practical-guide-designing-products-services-people-affected-dementia

Fleming, R., & Bowles, J. (1987). Units for the confused and disturbed elderly: Development, design programming and evaluation. *Australian Journal on Ageing, 6*(4), 25–28.

Fleming, R., Bowles, J., & Mellor, S. (1989). Peppertree lodge some observations on the first fifteen months of the first C.A.D.E. unit. *Australian Journal on Ageing, 8*(4), 29–32. https://doi.org/https://doi.org/10.1111/j.1741-6612.1989.tb00779.x

Gan, D. R. Y., Chaudhury, H., Mann, J., & Wister, A. V. (2021). Dementia-friendly neighbourhood and the built environment: A scoping review. *The Gerontologist.* https://doi.org/10.1093/geront/gnab019

Gordon, A., Burton, J., Everard, L., & Philippe, M. (2016). *Guidelines for the development of dementia-friendly communities.* https://www.dementia.org.au/sites/default/files/WA/documents/DFC-Guidelines%20Doc%20Final.pdf

Gutman, G. M. (1989). *Dementia patients in institutions: A review of recommendations and research concerning their design, staffing and programming needs* [Book]. Gerontology Research Centre, Simon Fraser University, Vancouver, B.C. https://proxy.lib.miamioh.edu/login?url=https://search.ebscohost.com/login.aspx?direct=true&db=gnh&AN=52473&site=ehost-live&scope=site

Halsall, B., & MacDonald, R. (2017). *Design for Dementia: Vol 1- A Guide* (Vol. 1). TheHalsall Lloyd Partnership. https://www.hlpdesign.com/images/case_studies/Vol1.pdf

Hiatt, L. (1985, November 12-15). *Designing for mentally impaired persons: Integrating knowledge of people with programs, architecture and interior design.* American Association of Homes and Services for the Aging Annual Conference, Los Angeles, CA, United States.

Hiatt, L. G. (1980). Disorientation is more than a state of mind. *Nursing Homes, 29*(4), 30–36.

Hiatt, L. G. (1980). The happy wanderer. *Nursing Homes, 29*(2), 27–31.

Hiatt-Snyder, L., Rupprecht, P., Pyrek, J., Brekhus, S., & Moss, T. (1978). Wandering. *The Gerontologist, 18*(3), 272–280.

Judd, S., Marshall, M., & Phippen, P. (1998). *Design for dementia.* Journal of Dementia Care, Hawker Publications Ltd.

Karr, A. (1849). *Les Guêpes*, 'The Wasps' (a monthly pamphlet), reprinted in Vol. 6 (1891) of the collected series, 305.

Keen, J. (1989). Interiors: Architecture in the lives of people with dementia. *International Journal of Geriatric Psychiatry, 4*, 255–272.

Krier, D., de Boer, B., Hiligsmann, M., Wittwer, J., & Amieva, H. (2023, July 1). Evaluation of dementia-friendly initiatives, small-scale homelike residential care, and dementia village models: a scoping review [Review Article]. *Journal of the American Medical Directors Association, 24*(7), 1020–1027. https://doi.org/10.1016/j.jamda.2023.03.024

Lawton, M. P. (1986). *Environment and aging* (2nd ed., Vol. Series I, Vol. I). Center for the Study of Aging.

Lawton, M. P., & Nahemow, L. (1973). Ecology and the aging process. In C. Eisdorfer & M. P. Lawton (Eds.), *Psychology of adult development and aging.* American Psychological Association.

Liebowitz, B., Lawton, M. P., & Waldman, A. (1979a). Evaluation: Designing for confused elderly people. *American Institute or Architects Journal, 68,* 59–61.

Liebowitz, B., Lawton, M. P., & Waldman, A. (1979b). A prosthetically designed nursing home. *American Institute of Architects Journal, 21,* 88–98.

Mace, N., & Rabins, P. V. (1981). *The 36-hour day.* The Johns Hopkins University Press.

Marquardt, G., Buetter, K. & Motzek, T. (2014). Impact of the design of the built environment on people with dementia: An evidence-based review. *Health Environments Research & Design Journal, 8*(1), 127–157.

Nowak, S. J. M., Molema, C. C. M., Baan, C. A., Oosting, S. J., Vaandrager, L., Hop, P., & De Bruin, S. R. (2015). Decentralisation of long-term care in the Netherlands: the case of day care at green care farms for people with dementi. *Ageing and Society, 35*(4), 704–724. https://doi.org/10.1017/S0144686X13000937

Pozo Menéndez, E., & Higueras García, E. (2022, October 31). Best practices from eight European dementia-friendly study cases of innovation. *International Journal of Environmental Research and Public Health, 19*(21). https://doi.org/10.3390/ijerph192114233

Pritchard, R. J. (1990). "Better way" to care for dementia sufferers. *Ageing International, 16*(1), 44–46. https://proxy.lib.miamioh.edu/login?url=https://search.ebscohost.com/login.aspx?direct=true&db=gnh&AN=51658&site=ehost-live&scope=site

Richmond, D. T. (1983). *Inquiry into Health Services for the Psychiatrically Ill and Developmentally Disabled: Report Recommendations Summary.*

Schmachtenberg, T., Monsees, J., & Thyrian, J. R. (2022, November 18). Structures for the care of people with dementia: A European comparison. *BMC Health Services Research, 22*(1), 1372. https://doi.org/10.1186/s12913-022-08715-7

Schultz, D. (1987). Special design considerations for Alzheimer's facilities. *Contemporary Long Term Care Journal* 10 (11), 48–56, 112.

Wu, S.-M., Huang, H.-L., Chiu, Y.-C., Tang, L.-Y., Yang, P.-S., Hsu, J.-L., Liu, C.-L., Wang, W.-S., & Shyu, Y.-I. L. (2019). Dementia-friendly community indicators from the perspectives of people living with dementia and dementia-family caregivers. *Journal of Advanced Nursing, 75*(11), 2878–2889. https://doi.org/https://doi.org/10.1111/jan.14123

Zeisel, J., Bennett, K., & Fleming, R. (2020). *World Alzheimer Report 2020: Design, dignity, dementia: Dementia-related design and the built environment.* London, England: Alzheimer's Disease International. https://www.alzint.org/resource/world-alzheimer-report-2020/

3

Advances in research and practice on environmental design of care facilities for people living with dementia

Kevin Charras

Background

Some might think that research on environmental design for people living with dementia almost ceased, with fewer studies on environmental design models published over the past years. After all, what remains to change, once we have defined the environmental dimensions for architectural design for people with dementia? Research is characterized by different phases and some of these are perhaps less creative and/or productive than others, but are essential, nonetheless. The COVID-19 pandemic led decision-makers and experts around the world to question the very concept of nursing homes and long-term care facilities and, of course, the way that people living with dementia were taken care of in these settings. The history of thinking about design for dementia is characterized by different models or approaches, described in the following paragraphs in more detail.

Main architectural design models for people living with dementia in care facilities

Analysis of the literature on facility design for people living with dementia (PwD) yields five major models or approaches, which can be categorized as: (1) therapeutic, (2) rehabilitative or ergonomic, (3) needs-based, (4) experiential, and (5) use of space.

Therapeutic: Zeisel, Hyde, and Levkoff (1994) developed an integrative Environment-Behavior approach for PwD by combining the existing models of Calkins (1988), Cohen and Weisman (1991), Hiatt (1991), and Lawton (1987). This model is called *therapeutic,* because its initial basis lies in a mind-brain perspective, and it is geared to compensate for the cognitive losses seen in dementia.

Rehabilitative or ergonomic: Marshall (1998) and Fleming and Pundare (2010) posited that the goal of their combined design guidelines was to compensate for cognitive and physical disability and to maximize independence of residents with dementia. Because this model focuses on overcoming deficits by using environmental design, we refer to it as *ergonomic* or *rehabilitative.*

DOI: 10.4324/9781003416241-5

Needs-based: Morgan and Stewart's (1999) model can be designated as being *needs-based,* because they base their recommendations on an approach relating to the needs of the residents within a Person-Environment (P-E) interaction perspective. Implementation of their recommendations was intended to decrease challenging behaviors, which reflect discontent of PwD by meeting their needs.

Experiential: Davis et al. (2009), in an approach that could be referred to as *experiential,* stress the need to shift from 'condition' to 'experience' in order to "facilitate the culture change needed to create environments that allow the person with dementia to be an active participant in everyday life rather than a passive recipient of care" (p. 186–187).

Use of space: Charras, Eynard, and Viatour (2016) propose a conceptual framework that emphasizes the necessity of examining the *use of space* when designing living environments for PwD to enable behavioral settings to fit social, cognitive, and psychological competences of its users and directly refer to underlying human rights triggered by architectural design. The authors posited that a conceptual framework relying on human-environment transactions has a better chance of fitting with cultural differences as well as individual preferences rather than a design model based on single cultures.

These models have been implemented in a number of long-term care facilities and have received significant attention from stakeholders. However, there has been no scientific consensus for preference of use for any of these models, although some have been implemented internationally. Several reasons can be identified, amongst which lack of evidence seems to be central.

Evidence-based architectural design

Evidence-based architectural design for people with dementia is an Eldorado that is not always attainable. A number of studies have suggested that adapted design has positive outcomes on quality of life of people with dementia, but these were also confronted by the methodological difficulties in isolating environmental variables that effectively do so. To our knowledge, only one study managed to retrospectively assess an inventory of environmental design features of 15 special care units and associate these with behavioral health measures in 427 residents using a hierarchical linear modeling statistical technique (Zeisel et al., 2003).

Several lab-based research studies have shown positive results on how architectural design could improve skills in PwD, such as orientation in specific environments, for example. But very few studies, if none, have managed to show scientifically how living environments could enhance quality of life, activities of daily living, or relieve the behavioral and psychological symptoms of dementia, according to evidence-based research standards (Harrison et al., 2022).

The Cochrane Data Base has proceeded with a systematic meta-analysis of studies and evidently has drawn the conclusion – like it has for most nonpharmacological interventions – that there was insufficient proof to show effectiveness of architectural design to improve care for people with dementia (Harrison et al., 2022). However, what is observed empirically does not necessarily reflect the research results selected by the Cochrane review.

Such outcomes can question the veracity of empirical observations, or the epistemological grounds of evidence-based design as addressed by scientists. In the second case, we can argue that many research studies have shown evidence of the impact of design on dementia-related indicators using qualitative and quantitative methods which were identified as unfit with Cochrane review requirements.

The Cochrane review conclusions do not mean that research done in this area is flawed when designing facilities for people living with dementia. It mostly points out that we need grounded research with adapted epistemological means to evaluate the impact of environment on people living with dementia. In addition, it also points out the need to precisely define the objectives of designed environments in order to evaluate appropriate outcomes. It is possible that the different models used to design facilities combined in the Cochrane meta-analysis could have expected different outcomes, and thus should not have been combined in one meta-analysis. It thus seems inevitable to have to analyze different schools of thought that have emerged from architectural design of care facilities for people living with dementia.

From healing to inclusion

Architectural models discussed earlier in this chapter have built environmental responses congruently with care approaches, to attain desired behavioral goals.

Four philosophical mainstreams can be identified when analyzing these models: (i) equality, (ii) equity, (iii) prevention, and (iv) inclusion. Each of these approaches reflects societal evolutions and demands consideration of environments through different lenses to achieve different behavioral goals. Although previously exposed models have evolved through time and are not so clearly demarcated, they find their roots in each of these approaches (Figure 3.1):

1 Equality echoes with the rights of different groups of people to receive the same treatment. With this aim environmental design seeks to achieve therapeutic goals in order to heal symptoms and for people to gain equal dispositions to lead their life. Therapeutic environments are designed in such a way that its features are elaborated to relieve behavioral symptoms and enable equal opportunities for everyone.
2 Equity reflects situations in which everyone is treated fairly according to their needs. This approach naturally led to conceive environments with an ergonomic approach, in order to compensate for deficits and to

provide the same opportunities to each person. Environments originating from this angle are often acknowledged as "friendly environments": they enable people to access and use their environment in an equitable way. Ergonomic environments will pay attention to each person's abilities and structure the environment in a way that will lead them to use their environment in a standard manner.

3 Prevention is intended to stop something before it happens and in the field of health this is done to prevent diseases by avoiding unhealthy behaviors. Preventive design approaches were directly inspired from health promotion, from which salutogenesis holds its roots (Aantonovsky, 1996). Salutogenic design focuses on factors that support human health and well-being by encouraging people to maintain timely abilities (Golembiewski, 2022).

4 Inclusion is probably the most contemporary mainstream. It suggests that people living with dementia also have the right to age in place by maintaining independence and autonomy, connecting to social support, networks, and community, and encountering cultural, generational, and human diversity. Inclusion is about providing resources so that everyone can express their abilities to lead their life independently. Inclusion aims to design empowering and engaging environments that lead people to take control over their lives whatever needs they may express. Empowering environments mainly focus on how to trigger affordances and capabilities of people in order for them to lead a life congruently with their competences and expectancies.

These philosophical mainstreams do not deal with interactional and transactional people-environment relationships in the same way. Both interactional and transactional frameworks consider individual and contextual characteristics. The interactional framework suggests that environmental variables impact individuals with predisposed psychological traits and cognitive abilities in a deterministic way, whereas the transactional framework does not consider the individual as being merely passive and suggests that congruency between the person and the environment is modeled and processed by continuous transactions in which behaviors are modified by environment and conversely.

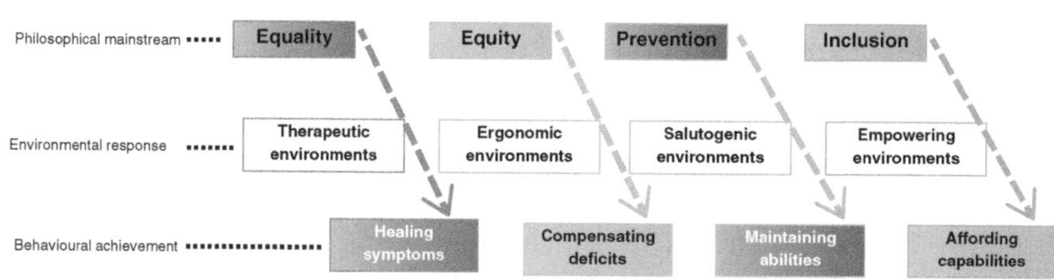

Figure 3.1 Philosophical mainstreams of residential care architecture for people living with dementia.

Equality and equity approaches are mostly driven by clinical concerns and focus on interactions between the environment and targeted behavior and abilities. Whereas prevention and inclusion approaches are driven by health and empowerment issues and focus on people-environment transactions until congruency between the two is reached.

Tom Kitwood's person-centered care (PCC) dimensions (attachment, identity, occupations, comfort, and inclusion; see Kitwood & Bredin, 1992) are fundamental to these mainstreams. Each dimension enables addressing the person and his/her relationships to the environment as a central piece in the design process. In addition, approaching the person with PCC involves addressing ethical perspectives in the field of care. Part of the responses to epistemological concerns on evidence-based design could be source of inspiration and trigger future research from this perspective.

Ethics, inclusion, and empowerment

While it may not seem straightforward, ethics can be a relevant way to untangle some of the concerns we have highlighted throughout this chapter. Some attempts have already been implemented in this vein. Charras, Eynard and Viatour (2016), for example, attempted to develop a framework for designing care facilities through the lenses of Human Rights. The reason for this choice was that Human Rights are universal and that people living with dementia remain citizens.

Some would refer to medical ethics to address the field of care facilities (beneficence, non-maleficence, autonomy, and justice). But a less normative and larger field, which relates to daily life, including empowerment and adjacent social relationships could be more adequate. Approaches described above all pay particular attention to the person's characteristics and singularity. Ethics of care is thus a meaningful angle to be used to regard the environmental design of care facilities for people living with dementia.

According to the Internet Encyclopedia of Philosophy ethics of care implies "moral significance in the fundamental elements of relationships and dependencies in human life". In addition to the ethical grounds it relies on, care as a practice relates specifically to meeting the needs of ourselves and others, thus referring to continuous transactional processes. From this angle, architecture's goal is to meet the needs of its users and more specifically the need of care processes whether referring to health or daily care. It should thus encourage the establishment of interdependent and transactional relationships between caregivers and care-receivers.

Such consideration leads us to precisely define the objectives of designed environments, in order to evaluate appropriate outcomes. Does architecture directly impact skills and competencies of its recipients? In which case architecture itself could be considered as therapeutic. Or, is it the use that is made of architecture and its consecutive transactions with users that will lead its recipients to adopt adaptive behaviors?

Proof of care: suggestion of an epistemological ground for evaluating residential care architectural design

Scientific evaluations of the impact of architecture on symptoms and well-being of people living with dementia do not meet gold standards of evidence-based science as defined by medical sciences (Harrison et al., 2022). However, multiplication and recurrence of similar observations tend to provide empirical evidence that there is an effect.

High co-occurrence of similar clinical observations should lead us to reconsider their generalizability and their possible qualification as *proof of care* (Fleury-Perkins & Fénoglio, 2019; 2022), by analogy to *proof of concept*. Proof of care could thus give indications of effectiveness, relevance, and maturity of experimental forms of residential care architecture and its correlation with clinical, therapeutic, resilient, and care attributes.

From this perspective, epistemological grounds of ethics of care (caring about, taking care, care-giving, and care receiving; Tronto, 1998) could serve as *proof of care* in order to evaluate residential care architecture through a 4-step approach as a prerequisite to traditional evidence-based evaluation (Figure 3.2):

1 *Caring about* is associated with identification, recognition and definition of a need for care. Attention paid to the person or people is a key aspect of this step, and caregivers – nurses, medical doctors, psychologists, and assistant nurses – are central in identifying needs. They should be documented and clinically substantiated by:

- observations of caregivers and/or relatives;
- expression of a need on the part of the concerned person or people;
- social, societal, political, public health, organizational, and/or institutional incentives.

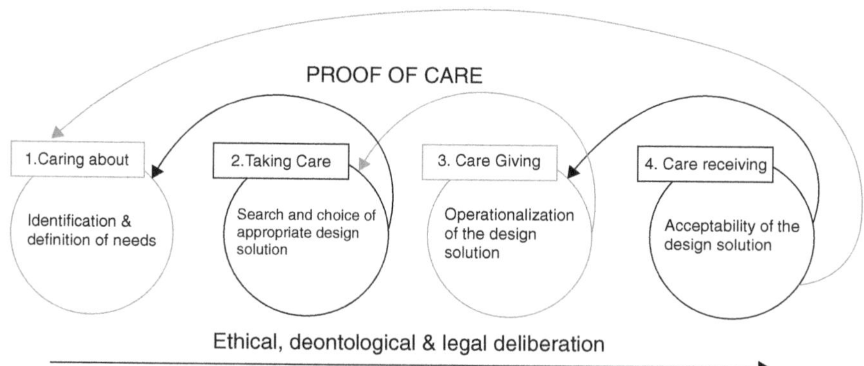

Figure 3.2 Processing steps of proof of care for residential care architectural design.

2 *Taking care* relates to taking responsibility for searching and choosing appropriate design solution(s). Solutions must be supported clinically and/or scientifically (theoretical framework, basic, clinical, and applied research) to substantiate its relevance to meet identified needs. The moral rationale of this step involves clinical responsibility of those who decide to implement it. Scientific and clinical literature can be a source of inspiration and argumentation for the choice of an architectural design solution. If no architectural design solution seems suitable or imaginable, this may mean that the definition of the need is incomplete or inaccurate to the person or the context.

3 *Care-giving* targets operationalization of the design solution in clinical practice. This phase requires investigating the possibility and feasibility of adapting the design solution to the clinical, institutional, organizational context, or conversely by adapting the context to the considered solution. It will be subject to specific consideration on the use of design features and its adequacy with deontological and ethical values of professional caregivers, and to a consultation with the recipients of the design solution.

Operationalization necessarily involves translating the imagined solution into practice in order to experiment and test it on a small scale. Observation or feedback reports (e.g., post-occupation evaluation) are shared and analyzed collectively with the entire care team. This phase constitutes proof of the feasibility of the envisaged innovation. Architectural design solutions can sometimes be experimented on a small scale and at low cost. If the operationalization does not seem appropriate, this may lead to reconsideration of the adequacy of the theoretical, clinical, and/or scientific framework.

4 *Care-receiving* concerns acceptability of the design solution within the framework of care relationships that should be established between the care effectors and receivers. The interdependence created by the design solution is directly targeted by congruency of actions and goals of caregivers with the demands of users. The search for the expected effect is obviously important, but what is central in this phase is the acceptability of the envisaged solution and the routine it engages by the protagonists of care. This phase is documented by patient and caregiver feedback. It can be supported and illustrated by quantitative or qualitative data from routine care on a test sample or by clinical case studies.

Feedback will also be an opportunity to strengthen ethical concern related to the tested solution. A solution that is unacceptable for patients or creates ethical dilemma for caregivers would indicate the need to reassess operationalization of the design solution.

These four steps are similar to those used in social design presented in three stages: inspiration-ideation-and implementation. In a general manner, recipients of the architectural design solution should be consulted at every step of the process; they take part in the elaboration and the evaluation phases (see Part 2 of this book : People with dementia are central to the design process). Ethical, deontological, and legal deliberations should be led along in the process to ensure appropriateness of the architectural design solution. The evaluation process is iterative in the sense that each phase requests to potentially revisit the previous one, and the last phase to revisit each of the three previous ones. Finally, it is "immersive" due to the need to implement architectural design solutions in the real world to observe what hinders and drives good care practices.

Proof of care evaluation process serves as a prerequisite in order to ensure that the goals of the architectural design solution are well reached before moving-on to evidence-based experimental methods. Proof of care can thus adjust to different residential care architecture mainstreams and help to identify appropriate indicators (scales, items, questions...) for future scientific evaluation.

Conclusion

Architectural trends for residential care of people living with dementia have followed philosophical mainstreams of care and have engaged in prolific and creative design solutions. However, research has sometimes failed to evaluate properly the solutions, due to lack of evidence. Architectural design cannot only rely on the ingenuity of architects and omit users from the design process.

Proof of care ensures that users (people living with dementia, caregivers, and family) take fully part in the elaboration and evaluation process of architectural design. Indeed, co-conception by involving users from the very beginning of architectural design of residential care homes is highly recommended (Nédélec, Somme & Charras, 2023). It helps stakeholders and policymakers to make the right choices, guarantees residents feel at ease with their environment and gives the opportunity to caregivers to practice in optimal conditions.

In-depth box

- We need grounded research with adapted epistemological means to evaluate the impact of environment on people living with dementia, and precisely define the objectives of designed environments, in order to evaluate appropriate outcomes.
- Five major dementia-specific design models can be identified in the literature: (1) therapeutic; (2) rehabilitative or ergonomic; (3) needs-based; (4) experiential; and (5) use of space.

- Philosophical mainstreams to which these specific design models respond may help to define the objectives of designed environments, in order to evaluate appropriate outcomes.
- High co-occurrence of similar clinical observations should lead us to reconsider their generalizability and their possible qualification as *proof of care* by analogy to *proof of concept*.

References

Antonovsky, A. (1996). The salutogenic model as a theory to guide health promotion. *Health promotion international*, 11(1), 11–18.

Calkins, M.P. (1988). *Designing for Dementia Planning: Environments for the Elderly and Confused*. Maryland: National Health Publishing.

Charras, K., Eynard, C., & Viatour, G. (2016). *Use of space and human rights: planning dementia friendly settings.* Journal of Gerontological Social Work. 59(3), 181–204. doi:10.1080/01634372.2016.1171268

Cohen, U., & Weisman, G.D. (1991). *Holding on to Home: Designing Environments for People with Dementia*. Baltimore, MD: Johns Hopkins University Press.

Davis, S., Byers, S., Nay, R., & Koch, S. (2009). *Guiding design of dementia friendly environments in residential care settings.* Dementia, 8(2), 185–203. doi:10.1177/1471301209103250

Fleming, R., & Purandare, N. (2010). *Long-term care for people with dementia: environmental design guidelines.* International Psychogeriatrics, 22(7), 1084–1096. doi:10.1017/S1041610210000438

Fleury-Perkins, C., & Fenoglio, A. (2019). *Le design peut-il aider à mieux soigner? Le concept de proof of care.* Soins, 64(834), 58–61.

Fleury-Perkins, C., & Fenoglio, A. (2022). *Ce qui ne peut être volé*. Charte du Verstohlen, Paris: Gallimard.

Golembiewski, J.A. (2022). *Salutogenic architecture.* In M.B. Mittelmark, G.F. Baueur, L. Vaandrager, J.M. Pelikan, S.Sagy, M. Eriksson, B. Lindström, & C.M. Magistretti (Eds.) *The Handbook of Salutogenesis 2nd edition* (259–274). Cham (Switzerland): Springer International Publishing.

Harrison, S. L., Dyer, S. M., Laver, K. E., Milte, R. K., Fleming, R., & Crotty, M. (2022). *Physical environmental designs in residential care to improve quality of life of older people.* Cochrane Database of Systematic Reviews, (3), Art. No.: CD012892. doi: 10.1002/14651858.CD012892.pub2.

Hiatt, L. G. (1991). Designing specialized institutional environments for people with dementia. In P.D. Sloane & L.J. Mathew (Eds.) *Dementia units in long-term care* (174-197). Michigan: Johns Hopkins University Press.

Kitwood, T., & Bredin, K. (1992). *Towards a theory of dementia care: personhood and well-being.* Ageing & Society, 12(3), 269–287.

Lawton, M.P. (1987). *Environmental approaches to research and treatment* of Alzheimer's disease. In E. Light & B. Liebowitz (Eds.) *Alzheimer's Disease, Treatment and Family Stress: Directions for Research*. Rockville, MD: National Institute of Mental Health.

Marshall, M. (1998). *How it helps to see dementia as a disability*. The Journal of Dementia Care, 6(1), 15–17.

Morgan, D.G., & Stewart, N.J. (1999). *The physical environment of special care units: needs of residents with dementia from the perspective of staff and family caregivers*. Qualitative Health Research, 9(1), 105–118.

Nédélec, P., Somme, D., & Charras, K. (2023). *L'architecture des Ehpad et son influence sur le bien-être des résidents*. Gérontologie et Société, 46(2), 105–124. doi:10.3917/gs1.171.0105

Tronto, J.C. (1998). *An ethic of care*. Generations: Journal of the American society on Aging, 22(3), 15–20.

Zeisel, J., Hyde, J., & Levkoff, S. (1994). *Best practices: an environment-behavior (E-B) model for Alzheimer special care units*. American Journal of Alzheimer's Care and Related Disorders and Research, 9, 4–21. doi:10.1177/153331759400900202

Zeisel, J., Silverstein, N. M., Hyde, J., Levkoff, S., Lawton, M. P., & Holmes, W. (2003). *Environmental correlates to behavioral health outcomes in Alzheimer's special care units*. The Gerontologist, 43(5), 697–711.

People with dementia are central to the design process

The voice of people with dementia at the core of environmental design

Emily Ong, Martin Robertson, Dennis Frost, Habib Chaudhury and Richard Fleming

> Accessible design cuddles and invites people of all abilities to explore and interact without feeling inadequate.
>
> – Emily Ong

The ability to maintain some level of independence, autonomy, and dignity is crucial to the quality of life experienced by people with dementia, regardless of the type and severity of their condition. The changes in the brain caused by the underlying diseases affect how people with dementia perceive, interpret, and interact with the environment. Over the last five years since Emily's diagnosis, she could see how her sensory and cognitive impairments have impacted her experiences of the places she visits. There are places that she used to enjoy going but now are out of bounds because of the disabling design of the built environment.

Dementia-enabling environmental design can compensate for some degree of the cognitive impairment faced by people with dementia. However, most dementia-friendly built environments are not planned and designed with insight from people living with dementia and more as a symbol of societal virtue. The development in inclusive and informed design decision-making has been slow, and only in the last decade has there been an emerging interest in environmental design for and with people with dementia as discussed in the next section.

Environmental design development (RF)

Since 2010, there have been four major reviews of the literature published on the relationship between environmental interventions and the behaviours and quality of life of people with dementia. The authors of these all took a systematic approach to identifying the best available evidence. The review published in 2010 looked at 57 articles, the latest, published in 2018, reviewed 127 articles on residential buildings alone, reflecting the growth of interest in research in this area.

DOI: 10.4324/9781003416241-7

The 2010 review (Fleming & Purandare, 2010) concluded that designers could be confident about the positive effect of unobtrusive safety measures, providing a variety of different rooms for different purposes, the provision of single rooms, controlling levels of stimulation, and providing good visual access so that residents can easily see the places that they want to go to.

The 2014 review (Marquardt et al., 2014) found that offering residents an environment that does not have an institutional design but has a homelike appearance and allows for individual transformations has positive effects on behaviour, well-being, social abilities, and care outcomes.

The 2017 review (Chaudhury et al., 2017) concluded that there is substantial evidence on the influence of unit size, spatial layout, homelike character, sensory stimulation, and environmental characteristics of social spaces on residents' behaviours and well-being in care facilities.

The 2018 review (Bowes & Dawson, 2018) highlighted the problems of separating out the impact of design features from that of care delivery on the quality of care, but the authors were able to conclude that, generally, homelike care homes are better, and design interventions can reduce levels of agitation, provide better opportunities for people to move about purposefully, and assist with improved communication between staff and residents.

The methodological problems highlighted by Bowes and Dawson must not be overlooked. Our research methods and tools, while improving, are still at a relatively early stage of development and do not perform well when compared to well-funded, medical model methodologies based on randomized trials, leading to some uncertainty about the results of the research (Harrison et al., 2022). However, despite the difficulties and uncertainties, there is a broad consensus emerging on the key characteristics of design that enable people living with dementia to fulfil their potential (Fleming et al., 2022). The emergence of this consensus is described in Chapter 16 of this book.

One of the critical areas of improvement is the emphasis being placed on the involvement of people with the lived experience of dementia being co-designers of the services and facilities that they use (Charras, 2020). But adoption of a co-design approach will have its challenges because discrimination against people with dementia is real and pervasive, as highlighted in the next section.

Designing for dementia rights

Globally, more than 55 million people live with dementia, and there are approximately 10 million new cases yearly. Dementia is one of the significant causes of disability, preventing many people from participating in social, cultural, and leisure life on equal terms with other citizens. Instead of finding ways to reduce the impact of disabilities on functioning and participation, people with dementia are kept behind locked doors in their own homes or in institutionalized care and are segregated from others, a treatment like convicted criminals (Swaffer, 2020).

The human rights and disability rights of people with dementia are often denied and violated despite the call for a human rights-based approach by the World Health Organization in 2015 at the First WHO Ministerial Conference on the Global Action Against Dementia. People with dementia have equal citizen rights (Bartlett & O'Connor, 2007) to participate fully and the right to live independently and be included in the community under the Convention of Rights for People with Disabilities (CRPD). People with dementia want to stay connected, engaged, and valued members of their communities.

When the architectural design has dementia rights at its core, it can help to improve the dignity, independence, and autonomy experienced by people with dementia. In 2020, Alzheimer's Disease International (ADI) launched the World Alzheimer's Report 2020 on "Design, Dignity, Dementia: Dementia-related design and the built environment" (Fleming et al., 2020), and called on governments to embed dementia design in their national dementia responses under the Convention on the Rights for Persons with Disabilities.

However, the response has been poor, and so far, initiatives such as the Dementia Friendly Communities have not made much meaningful impact on improving inclusion, and people with dementia continue to be disabled by the inaccessible built environment.

DAI environmental design special interest group (EDSiG)

In 2021, Dementia Alliance International (DAI), a registered U.S. non-profit 501 (c)(3) charity organization of, by, and for people with dementia, set up the Environmental Design Special Interest Group (DAI Website, 2021). The SiG functions as a community of practice to identify ways to support the implementation of the Design, Dignity, Dementia report by reaching out to community leaders, policymakers, and architectural and design associations, to get them to consider and implement inclusive, dementia-enabling environmental design to improve the quality of life for people with dementia (Ong et al., 2023).

EDSiG considers the environment to be more than the built environment; it encourages discussion on all aspects of the environment:

- Built environment – how can buildings and community infrastructures be designed in a manner that is accessible and usable by everyone, including people with cognitive disability?
- Social environment – how can a social environment in various contexts (e.g., neighbourhood, residential care setting, care environment) be intentionally generated and fostered to reflect the shared values of a community, reducing stigma, and facilitating inclusion?

- Rehabilitative and accessible environment – how can the environment reduce impairments impact, activity limitation, and participation restrictions? How can environments secure the human rights to be safe, included, and participate (guided by the Conventions of the Rights of Persons with Disabilities)?
- Transport and movement in the environment – how can environments support the ease of movement to meaningful people and places?
- Natural environment – how can we incorporate the natural surroundings to provide peace and tranquillity to the quality of life of those living with dementia who need the calmness from nature as a healing therapy?
- Technology in the environment - how can technologies support the inclusion and participation of people living with dementia?
- Sustainable environment – how can sustainable architecture be used to optimize daylighting, natural ventilation, and thermal management in care and residential environments; native landscaping; renewable energy systems, and recyclable building materials to reduce negative environmental impacts like pollution and economically more viable options for the LMICs to adopt?

The group is open to people living with dementia, care partners, and professionals interested in environmental considerations to support optimal functioning, promote independence, and foster a better quality of life for those living with dementia. Three of our dementia experts by lived experience have been working as co-designers, and their respective projects are featured in this chapter. However, co-design with dementia experts by lived experience is relatively new and researchers are still exploring suitable ways to meaningfully engaged people with dementia of varying abilities as discussed in the next section.

The practice of co-design with dementia experts by lived experience (HC)

The paradigm shift in seeing people with dementia as 'experts' of their experiences (Sleeswijk Visser et al., 2005) and consumers and designers (Fischer, 2002) is a recent movement. In co-design, the role of designers and researchers is to facilitate and support "experts" of their own experience with tools for ideation and solution expression (Sanders & Stappers, 2008), and they become central to the design process. Through the working partnership with experts by lived experiences, researchers and designers become more empathic, inclusive, and collaborative, which goes beyond their professional skill set. However, there is a general lack of clarity on the exact nature of engagement of people with dementia. It is important to understand that engaging people with dementia in a co-design process requires an appreciation of memory and cognition challenges and is taken into a well-considered participatory process. An empathic relationship is needed where people with dementia can speak and share openly with the designers and care partners, as in the KITE project, for example (Lindsay et al., 2012).

The DemSCAPE project focuses on identifying neighbourhood destinations considered significant by people with dementia and neighbourhood-built environment features relevant to their outdoor mobility, engagement, and social participation. The study utilized a co-design approach with 32 community-dwelling people living with mild dementia to moderate dementia or mild cognitive impairment from urban and suburban areas in Metro Vancouver and Prince George British Columbia, Canada. A mixed-methods approach was employed, including semi-structured sit-down and walk-along interviews; photo and video documentation and elicitation to enable experts with lived experience to express themselves. Wherever possible, an individualized and tailored approach was applied to modify the research methods to support the participation of people with dementia. Balancing challenge, safety, and comfort in interviews was an ongoing consideration, as some participants chose routes above their routine level of outdoor activity leading to exhaustion.

In this study, rigor was enhanced by utilizing a collaborative and iterative approach, including people with dementia from piloting equipment to ongoing debrief meetings for research team members to refine the walk-along procedure based on feedback from participants at the end of the walk-along. The study protocol was informed by seven factors which contributed to the rigor of this mixed-methods design employing novel technology with people with dementia:

1 Multiple sessions (four interviews) with each participant to help build rapport and facilitate in-depth exploration of the topic.
2 Data triangulation using different methods (i.e., structured questionnaire, semi-structured sit-down and walk-along interviews, photo, and video documentation).
3 Analytic triangulation through independent coding of data by different research team members.
4 Conducting regular debrief meetings within the team to provide peer support on substantive, procedural, methodological, and ethical issues encountered through data collection and analysis.
5 Leaving an audit trail by documenting steps taken in data collection and analysis through reflection journals maintained to record substantive, procedural, and reflexive notes from the field.
6 Memos to document the thought process behind coding and analytic decisions.
7 Eliciting participant feedback on methods during data collection, particularly the walk-along interview, to support ongoing refinement of data collection procedures (Padgett, 2012).

This DemSCAPE project builds on the goals of the DFC movement:

1 Eliminating the stigma surrounding dementia.
2 Spreading dementia awareness and education.
3 Empowering people to know their rights.
4 Enhancing people's engagement in the community.
5 Improving accessibility of spaces and services (Alzheimer's Disease International, 2015; World Health Organization, 2017).

It also reflects the philosophy by centring initiatives and activities on the meaningful engagement, full inclusion, and social participation of people living with dementia at all stages (Alzheimer's Disease International, 2015).

Co-design with dementia experts by lived experience is taking shape in Asia too, particularly in Japan, Taiwan, and Singapore. In Singapore, the "Find Your Way" project is a wayfinding initiative by SBS Transit, a local public transport provider, to help people with dementia find their way around in bus interchanges and MRT stations with greater ease and confidence. The project is the first of its kind in the local public transport nodes that involve segmenting the respective bus interchanges and MRT stations into distinct zones represented by a different coloured nostalgic mural and supported by color-coded directional floor arrows with corresponding murals that point the way to the respective boarding berths or station exits.

The dementia experts by lived experience are both consumers and designers in the co-design process where they provide their experience as commuters and creative ways to remove barriers to improve accessibility, inclusivity, and independent traveling experience. The selection criteria for involvement in the co-design process are limited to people with dementia who are using public transport independently. They are regarded as "lead customers" (Patricia Seybold, 2006) to represent and speak for others living with mild dementia who might be commuting independently by bus and train. Other than the initial first meeting with a technical expert, the co-design team comprises two persons with dementia, three SBS Transit project staff, two young artists, and a consultant from Dementia Singapore. It is a low-cost form of co-design that can be practiced in low-middle-income countries (LMICs).

In the next section, three of our dementia experts by lived experience – MR, EO and DF, narrated their involvement and what co-design means to them at individual level.

Examples of co-design at the local level Scotland – a public inconvenience: better toilets for inclusive travel (see Mathews et al., this volume for more information on this project)

After I (MR) was diagnosed with dementia, I was not sure what I was going to do with my time until I went into the local Alzheimer's Resource Centre and picked up a leaflet regarding research. The leaflet did not say what it was about, just gave a time for the meeting. My wife and I went along out of curiosity, and it turned out that it was into public toilets and how unsuitable they were for people with dementia. This was in 2017, and the main researchers wanted people with dementia to go around their local area and look at public toilets to see how accessible they were for people with dementia. However, having accessible toilets does not necessarily mean the toilets are suitable for differently abled people.

We live in a rural area, and it did not take long to find public toilets that had no disabled access and even public toilets that were locked in a busy tourist area. The next available ones were over half an hour's drive away. However, the worst example we found was at our local supermarket when one sat down you are opposite the door which has a full-length mirror which is most disconcerting, even for people without dementia.

After around six months, we gathered in Dundee to share our results and find a name for the project. I came up with the chosen title, "The Public Inconvenience," a play on the word as they were not at all convenient. We then took our Report to the Scottish Government Civil Servants in Edinburgh, where we put on a little Play to show how horrendous the situation is. I was also interviewed, which is available online (Robertson, 2020). One tangible success I know about is that the ferries from the Scottish mainland to the Orkney and Shetland Isles have altered their toilets to the extent that they now hoist for non-ambulant users.

I found the co-design experience fun, interesting, and a bit depressing as it showed how bad the environmental design around public toilets is. Covid-19 struck, and the discussions were moved online via Zoom and Teams, making it possible for me to continue with my passion even though I live far away from central Scotland. My experiences through this project made me want to do more co-design research. I call it, "Catnip to the brain," and it all started in my local supermarket's disabled toilet.

Singapore – find your way: wayfinding in bus interchanges and MRT stations

When I (EO) was diagnosed with young-onset dementia in 2017, my greatest fears and concerns were losing my independence and feeling 'imprisoned' by the environment (Ong et al., 2023). The ability to decide when I want to go out and how I choose to move around plays a significant role in defining my freedom and independence.

I enjoy taking the bus and train rides in Singapore because the public transport system is well-connected and reliable. Hence, I was thrilled to be invited into the project team as a dementia consultant by experience helping to make traveling by bus and train more accessible, safe, and inclusive for people with mild dementia and older people.

Unlike other co-design projects, the "Find Your Way" project is stakeholder-based and not led by a researcher. The dementia consultants by lived experience also provide technical knowledge on design principles related to signages and wayfinding based on resources from Dementia Services Development Centre (DSDC), University of Stirling. At the ideation stage, a concept walkthrough was created based on the stakeholder understanding of older commuters and the two dementia consultants who are also bus and train commuters. The team has also carried out an impact journey to analyse the different aspects that could influence and improve the commuting journey based on different touchpoints and the stakeholder's capacity. Initially, I felt a bit frustrated because we were not aware of the regulations on space usage, but I have learned to compromise on the next best available space for the wall mural so long as it achieves the objective.

I found the visualization experience useful in helping to make our needs and preferences of the size, colour combinations, and positioning of the image easier to be understood by other team members (Figure 4.1).

After working together for over two years, the team members became more knowledgeable of how people with dementia see and interpret their surroundings. They become more inclusive in their design thinking, and we felt good about ourselves because we can use our lived experience to benefit the community.

Australia – appeal to the land and environment court

In the 10 years since I (DF) was diagnosed with Semantic Frontotemporal Dementia, I have seen an increase in groups adopting some Dementia Enabling Design principles. Initially, no group requested any input from people living with dementia, and about five years ago, there was a growing interest in asking for input, but their request was tokenistic since they had already committed to the designs. This attitude has begun to change. Many groups are now seeking input to their designs early in their planning stages, and significant and important changes are occurring. Most of the groups I have worked with have been involved with Dementia Awareness campaigns that have laid groundwork for their 'enlightenment'. Slowly these principles of designing an environment to help rather than hinder people with dementia are being adopted by the broader community and not just some residential care facilities.

The highlight for me came when a commercial redevelopment was proposed for a site within my community and less than 100 meters from my home. As required by local government, this proposal was circulated to all the nearby residents asking for their comments. Many of the elderly people living nearby were very distressed with the proposed design but didn't have the skills needed to raise their concerns with the building authority. I was able to articulate both my objections and those of some of my neighbours to the Council. I made reference to Environmental Design Principles we all endorse and included a short video trying to illustrate the negative impact this proposal would have on 'green space'.

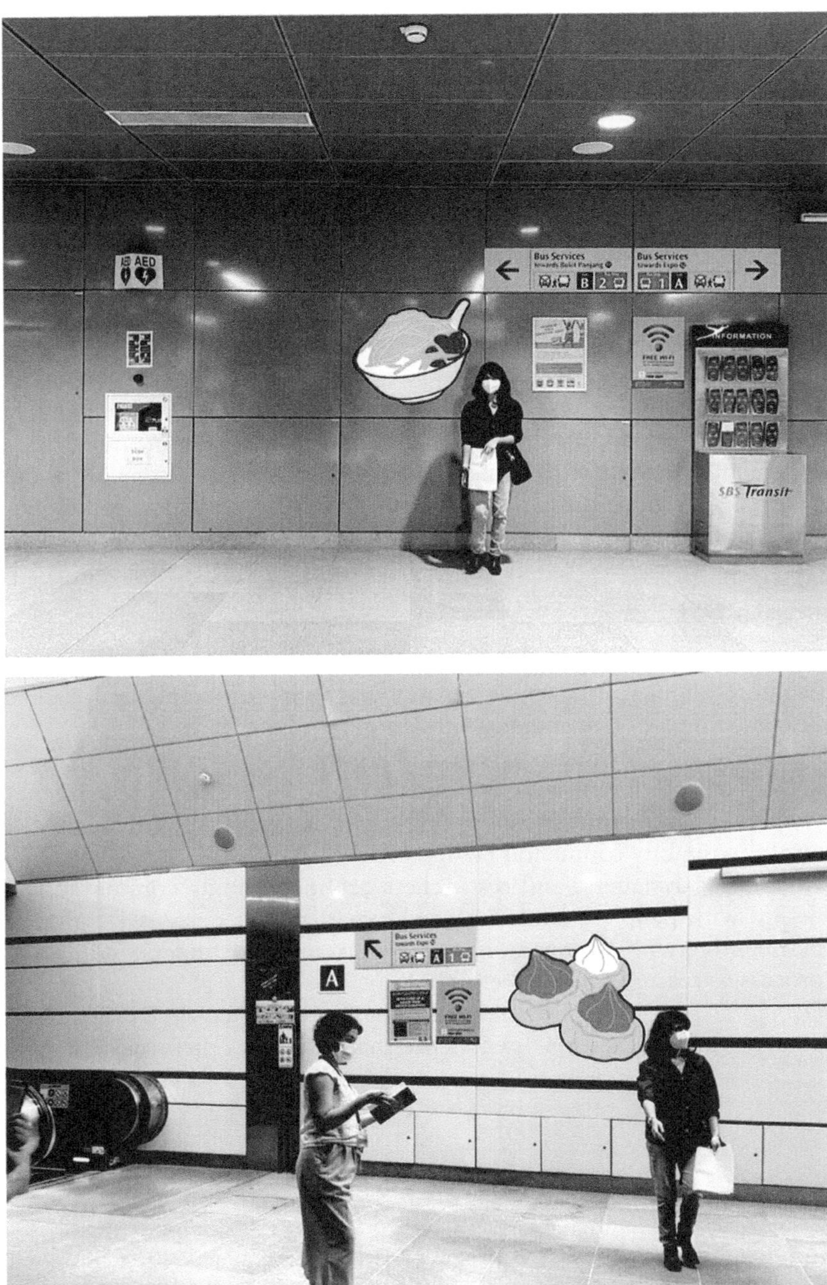

Figure 4.1 Visualization technique used in the wayfinding project. Photograph by the artist, Didier.

The result was that the council rejected this proposal. However, the commercial group behind it has appealed their decision to the 'Land and Environment Court'. The next step being an on-site hearing where I have been asked to state my case. To my knowledge, this is a first, at least locally if not nationally to have a person with lived experience put forward these principles at this level. Hopefully, I will have some good news soon and will be able to continue to walk within my local area with my head held high.

Summary

Co-design with dementia experts by lived experience is possible when technical experts including researchers are willing to be flexible and adaptive in their participatory approach. This chapter has clearly demonstrated that the involvement of people with dementia in the design process can contribute to better designs that address the needs of the people and their well-being as valued, contributing members of their community.

In-depth box

- There is a growing consensus on what constitutes enabling design that promotes dignity, independence, and autonomy for people with dementia discussed under environmental design development.
- There is a need for international collaboration between design professionals and people living with dementia to ensure that the human rights of people with dementia are always respected in the design process, which is a call by the Environmental Design SiG.
- Architects, designers, and researchers are increasingly committed to co-design with people having the lived experience of dementia and are experimenting with a range of approaches to improve understanding of this process as featured under DemSCAPE.
- Dementia experts by lived experience report that co-design is an enjoyable, stimulating learning experience that reinforces their sense of competence and worth as a person as stated by MR, EO, and DF.

References

Alzheimer's Disease International, *Dementia Friendly Communities (DFCs) New domains and global examples*. Alzheimer's Disease International, 2015. https://www.alz.co.uk/adi/pdf/dementia-friendly-communities.pdf

Bartlett, R., & O'Connor, D., 'From personhood to citizenship: broadening the lens for dementia practice and research'. *Journal of Aging Studies*, 21(2), 107–118, 2007. https://doi.org/10.1016/j.jaging.2006.09.002

Bowes, A., & Dawson, A., *Designing environments for people with dementia: a systematic literature review*. Emerald Publishing Limited, Bingley, UK, 2018.

Charras, K., Human rights, design and dementia: moving towards an inclusive approach. In Fleming, et al., *World Alzheimer Report 2020: design dignity dementia: dementia-related design and the built environment*, 2020. https://www.alzint.org/resource/world-alzheimer-report-2020/

Chaudhury, H., Cooke, H. A., Cowie, H., & Razaghi, L., The influence of the physical environment on residents with dementia in long-term care settings: a review of the empirical literature. *Gerontologist*, 58(5), e325–e337, 2018.

DAI Environmental Design Special Interest Group, 2021. https://dementiaallianceinternational.org/get-involved/special-interest-groups/ed-sig

Fischer, G., Beyond "couch potatoes": from consumers to designers and active contributors. *First Monday*, 7(12), 2002. https://doi.org/10.5210/fm.v7i12.1010

Fleming, R., Bennett, K. A., & Zeisel, J., Values and principles informing designs for people living with dementia—an emerging international consensus. *Journal of Aging and Environment*, 1–10, 2022. https://doi.org/10.1080/26892618.2022.2062806

Fleming, R., & Purandare, N., Long-term care for people with dementia: environmental design guidelines. *International Psychogeriatrics*, 22(7), 1084–1096, 2010. https://doi.org/10.1017/s1041610210000438

Fleming, R., Zeisel, J., & Bennett, K., Design dignity dementia: dementia-related design and the built environment. *Alzheimer's Disease International*, 2020. https://www.alz.co.uk/research/world-report-2020

Harrison, S. L., Dyer, S. M., Laver, K. E., Milte, R. K., Fleming, R., & Crotty, M., Physical environmental designs in residential care to improve quality of life of older people. *Cochrane Database of Systematic Reviews* (3), 2022. https://doi.org/10.1002/14651858.CD012892.pub2

Lindsay, S., Brittain, K., Jackson, D., Ladha, C., Ladha, K., & Olivier, P., *Empathy, participatory design and people with dementia*. CHI '12 Conference on Human Factors in Computing Systems, 2012.

Marquardt, G., Bueter, K., & Motzek, T., Impact of the design of the built environment on people with dementia: an evidence-based review. *HERD: Health Environments Research & Design Journal*, 8(1), 127–157, 2014. https://doi.org/10.1177/193758671400800111

Ong, E., Frost, D., Kuliga, S., Layton, N., & Liddle, J., Creating a consumer-driven global community of practice to support action within environmental design with people living with dementia: Assistive technology challenges and opportunities. *Brain Impairment*, 1, 2023. https://doi.org/10.1017/BrImp.2023.4

Padgett, D. (2012). *Qualitative and mixed methods in public health*. SAGE.

Robertson, M., *A public inconvenience project*. University of Edinburgh, 2020. https://youtu.be/lVQlJ5ngG-M?list=PLewGw1aBfLCg8EpjdeKn9btceYCwCnepO

Seybold, P. B. *Bathing your organization in real-time customer context*. Patricia Seybold Group, Boston, MA, 2006. https://www.customers.com/articles/bathing-your-organization-in-real-time-customer-context/

Sanders, E., B. N., & Stappers, P. J., Co-creation and the new landscapes of design. *CoDesign*, 4(1), 5–18, 2008. https://doi.org/10.1080/15710880701875068

Sleeswijk Visser, F., Stappers, P. J., van der Lugt, & Sanders, E. B.-N., Contextmapping: experiences from practice. *International Journal of CoCreation in Design and the Arts*, 1(2), 119–149, 2005.

Swaffer, K., Reframing dementia through the lens of human rights. In L. Steel, K. Swaffer, L. Philipson, & R. Fleming (Eds.), *Human rights for people living with dementia: an Australian anthology*. University of Technology, Sydney, 13–15, 2020.

World Health Organization, *World report on ageing and health*. World Health Organization, 2017. https://apps.who.int/iris/handle/10665/186463

5

The use of virtual reality to support participatory design processes in environmental design for cognitive change

Lesley Palmer, Martin Quirke, Junjie Huang and Judith Phillips

Introduction

Perceptions of ageing and how these are represented in public discourse can subject older people to prejudice and stereotype, framing them as frail and vulnerable, as well as being opposed to or unable to engage with new technologies. Yet, old age does not prevent the use of technology (Tacken et al., 2005) and older people, including people living with cognitive change, can offer helpful insights and provide valuable expertise by experience when included in designing the places and spaces they occupy.

Existing literature on the use of virtual reality (VR) for people with cognitive change such as mild cognitive impairment (MCI) or dementia has focussed on VR for assessment, therapeutic treatment and/or stimulation (Appel et al., 2021). While the potential for VR for other applications involving people living with dementia is recognised in the literature, this research remains in its infancy (Kim et al., 2019).

The two studies we shall discuss challenge age-based assumptions of older peoples interest in, and ability to engage with, modern digital technology, specifically VR. The aim of both studies was to explore the usability of fully immersive virtual reality (VR) systems as tools to support participatory design processes in the design of supportive housing models for people over 55 years old, including those with cognitive change. The connected projects occurred between 2020 and 2023 and were undertaken by a team of architects and social scientists at the University of Stirling. The first study, *Demonstrating Impact in Housing, Health and Social Care* (DIHHSC) was conducted remotely (during COVID-19 pandemic restrictions) whilst in the second project, Designing Homes for Health Cognitive Ageing (DesHCA), VR-based research was conducted primarily in-person.

This chapter has three objectives: (1) To summarise the two studies into the use of VR to support participatory design processes in environmental design for cognitive decline. (2) To discuss the opportunities of VR as a co-design tool amongst underrepresented groups and enable a full-scale immersive experience of architectural design projects that improve end-user contribution

DOI: 10.4324/9781003416241-8

to the design process. (3) To propose that immersive VR-supported co-design methodologies may help to advance research on environmental design for dementia in a global context.

We suggest there exists an opportunity to deploy VR in the design of the built environment to enhance the design process by engaging the views of underrepresented groups such as older people and people living with cognitive change through their expertise by experience. VR enables the participant to immerse themselves in the environment and experience deeper 'presence' (Kim et al., 2019) as opposed to observing in 2D either on a flat-screen or paper print-out. With the full scale, and hyper-realistic nature of VR offering improved kinaesthetic sensation, both studies examined the extent to which VR-supported experiences of design proposals provided 'enhanced ecological validity', compared with traditional paper-based approaches to design review (Manera et al., 2016). VR-supported experience and review of design provide a powerful means overcoming the barriers of reading or interpreting architectural drawings, and positively influence participants' abilities to provide a deeper, more informed critique of design. We suggest that design critique improves with greater immersion and environmental role-play.

Finally, we hypothesise that the use of VR remotely in a global context can assess the efficacy of dementia design principles by engaging international users remotely in future environmental design research projects, thus gauging suitability of design features in regional contexts.

Background

Environmental design for dementia

The research team has expertise in environmental design for people living with dementia; a recognised non-pharmacological intervention to ameliorate psychological behavioural symptoms of dementia (PBSD),[1] and are experienced in its application on capital development projects globally (Kiuchi et al., 2020; Palmer et al., 2021).[2] Environmental design for dementia or 'dementia-friendly' design principles have been in existence since the 1980s (Fleming & Bowles, 1987). Evolving from these design principles and the research evidence that support them (Bowes & Dawson, 2019; Fleming & Purandare, 2010) are several environmental assessment tools which provide design guidelines prescribing design features which when implemented contribute to a dementia-friendly environment. Examples include the Dementia Design Assessment Tool (Cunningham et al., 2008), Enhancing the Healing Environment (The King's Fund, 2014), the Environmental Audit Tool (Bennett & Fleming, 2013) and the Therapeutic Environmental Screening Survey (Sloane et al., 2002). There was, however, a dominant environment in early tools (the care environment) and this reflected the prevailing wider societal understanding of the environment in which people with dementia inhabited, i.e., long-term care and not within the community. Recognising that people with dementia live within community settings, more recent design tools seek to provide guidance on designing community spaces (Fleming et al., 2017; Henry et al., 2021).

More recently, research concerned with the generalisability of dementia design calls for critical discussion and new research to reflect global diversity, acknowledging that past research evidence has tended to reflect and reproduce the context of its production (Dawson & Palmer, 2020). The challenge to the delivery of dementia design in other cultures, countries and environment types is the need for those who are commissioning and designing environments to be familiar with overarching dementia-design principles. And further, to be sufficiently adept in their knowledge to be capable of suitably sensitive application of the principles to design and deploy environment features which are familiar to users whilst complementing the context of their application. Without this, the application of culturally imbued design features in another culture risks undermining the efficacy of the intervention.

It is important to note that a distinction is made by the authors between dementia-design principles and the features described in assessment tools and design guides. We favour the definition of 'design principle' as the overarching theme, and 'design feature' being the attribute which contributes to achieving the principle; most commonly the architectonic elements such as a door, chair or handle, and wall or floor finishes. This distinction is made in recognition that design principles, when considered in a global context, enable a more nuanced, culturally relevant approach to environmental design. Design features by contrast are specific; culturally imbued, influenced by the local vernacular, building codes and assume user familiarity.

Architectural design process and barriers

Conventional architectural design process is intricate and multifaceted, involving a series of activities that range from initial conceptualisation to project realisation. There are numerous barriers that can affect this process, including technical challenges, knowledge gaps and constraints imposed by the available communication tools (Kvan, 2000). Conventional design communication tools and methods such as sketches, 2D drawings, 3D models, blueprints, written reports and presentations, often fall short in conveying the full essence of the design, leading to misunderstandings and misinterpretations. Furthermore, these conventional methods can create an exclusionary process, whereby certain stakeholders, particularly those without specialised architectural knowledge, are inadvertently left out of the conversation.

Default othering

'Othering', as an effective conceptualised approach to learn emotional responses in medicine education (Shapiro, 2008) is also observed in the architectural profession (Buse et al., 2017). This concept refers to the tendency of architects to design based on their own perspective and anticipation of the end users. Such anticipation is built on 'imagined bodies' (Kerr, 2013) of the end users and knowledge gained from ideologies of care which reproduce prevailing ideals of care model and environment (Buse et al., 2017). It can be useful to reach an inclusive design result, but this can also result in environments that do not adequately consider the needs of diverse users. Such a 'default othering' approach often dominates the design process by its self-referential nature, leaving user experience and inclusion on the side lines. Lack of engagement with the actual end user has been one of the biggest challenges in architectural practice and becomes more problematic in designing for people living with dementia.

Conventional communication tools and methods in architectural design

Since the last decades of the 20th century, computer aided design (CAD) and building information modelling (BIM) emerged as a revolutionary tool in design, aiming to address some of these concerns. The CAD- and BIM-driven design approach allows for rapid prototyping and scenario testing, which can enhance the efficiency, productivity, quality and collaboration in construction workforce; an ethos advocated by Egan (1998) and Latham (1994). It centralises information, improving communication and understanding among project participants. However, CAD and BIM have their limitations. The primary concern is its accessibility, as the high cost of CAD and BIM software and necessary training often poses a barrier for non-professional end users, as well as smaller firms and individual architects (Succar, 2009). Moreover, the CAD and BIM process tends to focus heavily on technical and functional aspects of a building, sometimes overlooking the emotional, cognitive and sensory experiences of the end users. These concerns bring the question, where are the end users of design in these new tools? CAD, BIM and other similar technologies need to extend beyond the tangible and functional attributes of design and consider the experiential and human-centric aspects of architecture.

Recent advances in VR and related digital technology offer promising opportunities in this regard. VR allows designers to immerse themselves and their clients in the virtual representation of their designs, facilitating a better understanding of space, scale and user experience (Cousins, 2017; Portman et al., 2015). Moreover, VR has been used to simulate the experience of various user groups, such as individuals with disabilities, memory loss and dementia (Christie, 2017; Shen, 2021; Shen et al., 2021), thereby fostering empathetic and inclusive designs (Riva et al., 2021). These new technologies open another gate to designers and architects for user participation in inclusive design by experiencing and testing their ideas in VR. User participation could reduce the impact of gaps in designer knowledge, or flaws in their societal ideologies, helping to minimise othering during the design process.

House 1: Version 1

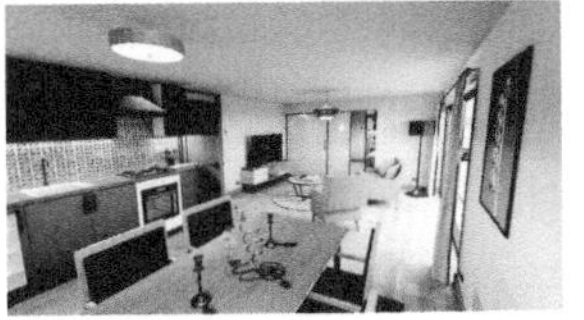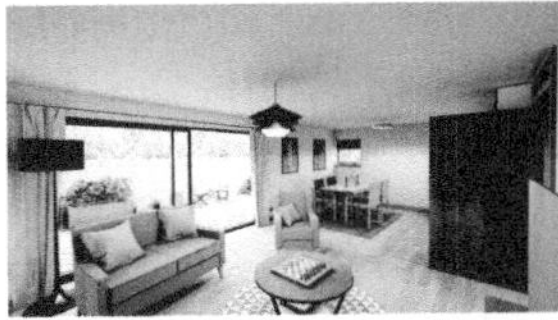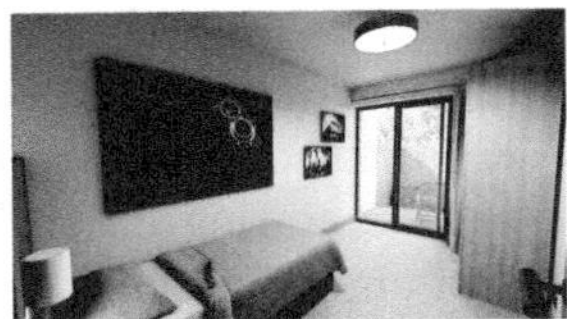

House 1: Version 3

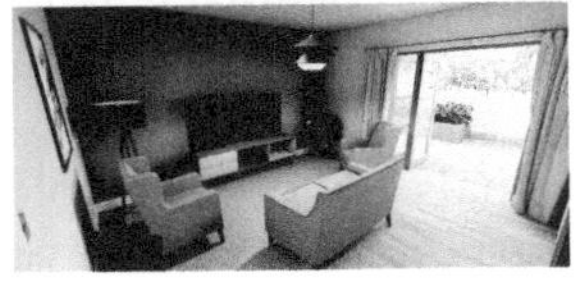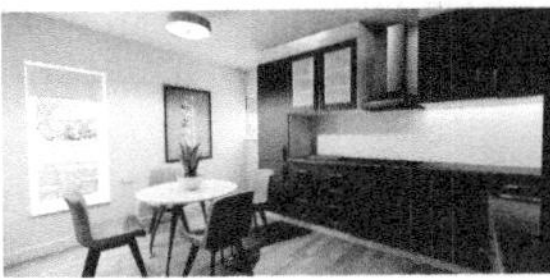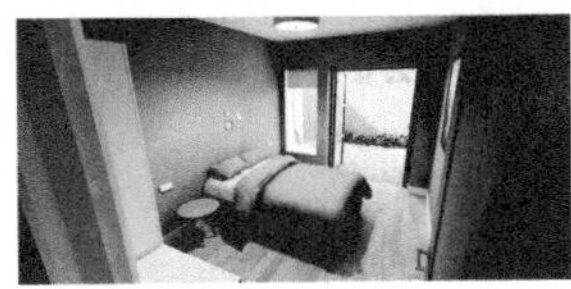

Figure 5.1 Virtual homes development in the case study projects.

VR and digital technology opportunities

VR is widely associated with recreational activities including gaming and has had success as a therapeutic tool to ease symptoms associated with conditions such as autism (Maskey et al., 2019), dementia (Appel et al., 2021) and post-traumatic stress disorder (Kothgassner et al., 2019). It is increasingly used as means of gamifying training, being especially useful for situations that are difficult to replicate in real life, due to cost, safety or perceptual reasons (Grassini & Laumann, 2020). More recently, the capability of VR to emulate audio visual and spatial perception challenges associated with conditions such as sight loss, hearing loss and dementia has allowed VR to provide immersive experiences that can enhance empathy towards people living with these conditions (Zwoliński et al., 2020). This chapter discusses two research studies that evidence a further constructive use of VR to support the meaningful involvement of people living with cognitive change in the architectural design process.

Experimental approach

Both studies revolved around the use of VR to support co-design of age and cognitively supportive homes. Both used iterative design processes, where protype home designs were improved and refined in stages (see Figure 5.1), in response to multiple rounds of participant feedback.

The first, and smaller, of the two studies, DIHHSC, was undertaken during national lockdowns associated with the COVID-19 pandemic. This necessitated a series of technical and methodological changes that would allow the research to proceed with remotely located participants. VR headsets were sent by courier to the participants homes, who were all older people living in various locations across England and Scotland. Participation took place over recorded MS Teams calls, where the researchers remotely guided participants through the virtual homes, prompting them for feedback on the designs.

The second and larger follow-up study, DesHCA, reverted to a face-to-face VR workshop format. This typically involved participants being supported on a one-to-one basis, by a member of the research team, as they experienced and commented on the VR home designs. Participants then joined facilitated group discussions about their experience of the VR. In this study, participants were a mixture of older people experiencing cognitive change and housing-related professionals, such as architects, builders and council officers.

Amongst the two participant sub-groups, professionals and older people, few older people reported having any previous experience of direct involvement in the environment design process. By contrast, many of the housing-related professionals contributed to design processes on a regular basis. Whilst some older people had been exposed to domestic adaptation or renovation projects in the past, only those with previous training in built environment disciplines admitted they could confidently understand or interrogate conventional design communication methods such as architectural floorplan drawings.

Participants exposure to, and confidence in using technology varied widely; from those who did not own or use a computer or smartphone through to those who were competent and confident users of internet-connected technologies such as smart speakers and social media.

Most participants were aware of VR and its use for gaming, but they had never previously experienced VR for themselves. Some participating housing professionals had previous recreational experiences of using VR, while only a handful indicated using it as part of an environmental design project. Even though the professionals contributing to the research included architects from firms who are known for co-creative design practices, none indicated any previous use of VR for end-user consultation or co-design processes.

The immersive nature of VR raised various questions around maintaining comfort, safety, and inclusion for participants of different abilities. This included concerns about risk of injury should the participant trip, or physically crash into objects whilst inside the headset. Similarly, that individuals may be uncomfortable wearing the VR headset, or potentially feel unbalanced or dizzy from the novel sensory experience. These issues were carefully considered in the design of the methods used for the research, which were approved by the University research ethics panel.

The VR headset-based activities took place in defined obstacle free spaces, making use of a digital boundary function, which provided visual warning to the users when they got close to the edge of a defined 'play' zone. One-to-one support provided by researchers helped participants to stay safe and comfortable during in-person workshops. For the remote workshops, ensuring that the participant's web camera was set up to see the full extent of their 'play' zone, allowed researchers to provide verbal safety cues where needed. Where participants were uncomfortable or unable to wear a VR headset, researchers could act as a proxy by casting a live video feed from the VR headset to a display screen and following the participant's instructions on where to go and what to look at in each VR model. In the DesHCA study, participants were provided with further alternative means of reviewing the designs, including print outs, pre-recorded video walkthroughs and an interactive web-based 3D viewer.[3]

Discussion

Co-production

Designing environments for people living with dementia and their care partners requires a deep understanding of their unique experiences and challenges. Conventional collaboration in architectural design involves stakeholders contributing their expertise and perspectives in a sequential manner. This allows architects to gain insights into the lived experiences of people with dementia, fostering the creation of supportive spaces tailored to their unique needs (Fleming et al., 2017). However, while effective, it may not capture the full spectrum of the end user needs or preferences, particularly for people with cognitive change who may find it difficult to understand the design drawings and express their experiences and preference verbally.

VR technology provides an effective platform to facilitate co-production and involve these individuals in the design process. In both the studies, regardless of whether joining remotely or in-person, participants immersed themselves in the virtual homes and actively left comments on the design features they felt were positive, or conversely uncomfortable or difficult to use. From these comments, the facilitators, as designers, were able to make sense of what the priorities are in the home environment that could better support healthy cognitive living. The virtual homes were then updated based on these priorities. During the walkthrough process, both the participants and the facilitator initiate a discussion or enquiry. The conversations between the facilitator and the participant in the virtual environment were interactive and engaged, as natural as the conversation in a physical building.

Removing the barriers to engagement within the design process

As most participants had not previously experienced VR, there was a sense of curious, yet nervous, excitement amongst them in advance of their VR experience. This feeling was more obvious amongst some participants who made statements like "I'm not much good with technology". However, in most cases, once participants put the VR headset on, they immediately began to enjoy the experience, typically becoming engrossed in the hyper-reality of what they were experiencing.

Within a few minutes of entering the VR, most participants had settled into the experience and were confidently navigating their way around the virtual environment, providing critique of the design. As the session progressed, and participants became more comfortable in their conversation with the researcher, they increasingly engaged in self-advocacy by providing rationale for observational feedback on the designs. This feedback linked to practical matters, personal taste, experience of caring for others or their personal experience of living with physical, sensory or cognitive impairments.

The alternative paper-print and screen-based methods for viewing the designs became valuable tools for supporting participant engagement in the research. In some cases, for more hesitant participants these mediums provided familiar initial ways of engaging with the designs, typically becoming steppingstones in building up confidence before later trying the full VR experience.

These mediums were also useful for the small number of participants who found the headsets uncomfortable for any reason. Reverting to the alternative viewing methods allowed these participants to maintain enjoyment of their participatory experience and contribution to the research. Notable differences for this group included that they made fewer observations overall, with their feedback containing reduced content or nuance around detailed design, especially spatial ergonomics, compared to participants who had reviewed the home designs in full VR.

Remote engagement & wider inclusion

The remote methodology of DIHHSC demonstrated the usability of VR for effective and efficient remote consultation with older people and people with cognitive decline. This has many potential future uses and we propose one wider application of this method could be use within resident/patient consultations in rural settings. For example, trialling a virtual home adaptation prior to construction whilst at the same time supporting the user to make informed decisions about their home and explore the appropriateness of the proposed adaptations. The remote methodology also presents wider implications for global research, which we discuss later.

DesHCA demonstrated the value that multi-disciplinary stakeholder consultation can bring. When stakeholders can engage on an equal standing in a fully immersive environment (i.e., without reliance on prior professional knowledge or experience to interpret paper-based architectural drawing) their confidence and ability to critique from their own experienced position improved.

Participant VR engagement in both studies enabled a form of 'process architecture' (Fröst & Warren, 2007), supporting collaborative engagement whereby ideas and expertise by experience were able to be tested, validated and incorporated as the design developed. This shifted the architectural process away from the linear approach of staged refinement (RIBA, 2020) to an iterative design-experience-design loop reconfiguring the design until a majority consensus was achieved, or no further changes proposed. This facilitated more detailed design critique and offered stakeholders greater exposure to and improved understanding of each other's needs.

The hyper-realism of the house designs and virtual environment in both studies, resulted in participants engaging in virtual 'house-play' (mimicking familiar activities – such as navigating a kitchen set-up within the virtual environment to assess the design suitability) whilst simultaneously providing design feedback/critique. This simultaneous experience-critique relationship demonstrated a high level of immersion and deep sense of presence within the virtual environment which researchers attributed to the quantity and depth of design comments received.

Wider implications on environmental design (principles) for dementia in other countries and cultures

The relationship between environments and culture is congruent; environments are cultured[4] (Rapoport, 1980). Environmental design is therefore variable, informed by the beliefs and behaviours of the culture in which it is located but conversely it also has a role in shaping and informing behaviours through its design. The central concern of environmental design for dementia in a global context is its suitability and applicability given the occidental cultural influence which informed the principal schema (Marshall, 2001). We suggest therefore that there is a conceptual approach made available through the development of our methodology. This methodology, especially with its geographically unrestricted remote participating functionality, can enable one to look globally at the dementia-environment interaction and role of 'culture' in the field of environmental design for dementia.

Conclusion

Two VR participatory co-design studies were undertaken between 2019 and 2023 with older adults with and without cognitive change. The studies demonstrated that older people can engage with VR for the first time, remotely, confidently and to such extent that their depth of presence within the virtual environment enables detailed, nuanced design critique. The hyper-realism and virtual-house play demonstrated that VR can equalise stakeholder engagement in the design process, providing a more balanced, equitable consultation and design process. Finally, the findings show that remote participatory co-design with VR can be successfully deployed over substantial geographic distance, enhancing the potential role for VR both within industry as a means of enhancing the process of environmental design for dementia, and as a means of supporting further advancement in participatory design research.

In-depth box

- Designing for dementia requires deep understanding unique experiences and challenges of the condition, but this is often absent from the design process.
- VR technology provides an effective platform for high quality co-production by supporting direct and meaningful end-user involvement in the design process.
- The hyper-realism of the immersive VR experience of design proposals, paired with verbalised experience-critique can significantly enhance the confidence, depth and nuance in stakeholder feedback on design proposals.
- Our VR supported participatory design methodology, including its remote participation functionality, is globally relevant, providing opportunities for improving environmental design for dementia across all cultures, locations and environment types.

Acknowledgements

The DIHHSC project was funded as part of the Escalator Fund of CHERISH-DE (Grant No. 30E) by the Engineering and Physical Sciences Research Council (EPSRC) in collaboration with the CHERISH-Digital Economy research centre at Swansea University. The DesHCA project was funded by the Economic and Social Research Council (ESRC), through the UK Research and Innovation (UKRI) Healthy Ageing Challenge: Social, Behavioural and Design Research (SBDRP) Programme. ESRC Grant Reference: ES/V016059/1.

Notes

1. https://www.stir.ac.uk/about/faculties/social-sciences/our-research/research-groups/cedar-centre-for-environment-dementia-and-ageing-research/
2. https://www.dementia.stir.ac.uk/
3. The VR design viewer used during participant workshops which was laterly overlaid with researcher design tips available at: https://www.deshca.co.uk/explore-deshcas-designs
4. For our purposes culture is the embodiment of a belief structure and lifestyle typical to one group.

References

Appel, L., Ali, S., Narag, T., Mozeson, K., Pasat, Z., Orchanian-Cheff, A., & Campos, J. L. (2021). Virtual reality to promote wellbeing in persons with dementia: A scoping review. *Journal of Rehabilitation and Assistive Technologies Engineering, 8*, 1–16. https://doi.org/10.1177/20556683211053952

Bennett, K., & Fleming, R. (2013). *The environmental audit tool handbook: DPD designing for people with dementia*. Dementia Training Study Centres. https://www.enablingenvironments.com.au/uploads/5/0/4/5/50459523/eat_handbook_july_13.pdf

Bowes, A., & Dawson, A. (2019). Designing environments for people with dementia. In *Designing environments for people with dementia* (pp. 1–92). Emerald Publishing Limited. https://doi.org/10.1108/978-1-78769-971-720191004

Buse, C., Nettleton, S., Martin, D., & Twigg, J. (2017). Imagined bodies: Architects and their constructions of later life. *Ageing and Society; Ageing and Society*, 37(7), 1435–1457. https://doi.org/10.1017/S0144686X16000362

Christie, J. (2017). Eyeing the possibilities of virtual reality. *Australian Ageing Agenda*, (May/June 2017), 52–53. https://search.informit.org/doi/10.3316/informit.018961122776310

Cousins, S. (2017, March 20). New tool to improve dementia design. *The RIBA Journal.* https://www.ribaj.com/products/living-with-dementia

Cunningham, C., Galbraith, J., Marshall, M., McClenaghan, C., McManus, M., McNair, D., & Pollock, R. (2008). *Dementia design audit tool* (1st ed.). University of Stirling.

Dawson, A., & Palmer, L. (2020). Environmental design education in a changing world. In R. Fleming, J. Zeisel, & K. Bennett (Eds.), *World Alzheimer Report 2020: Design dignity dementia: Dementia-related design and the built environment volume I* (pp. 208–217). Alzheimer Disease International. https://www.alz.co.uk/u/WorldAlzheimerReport2020Vol1.pdf

Egan, J. (1998). *Rethinking construction: The report of the construction task force.* HMSO.

Fleming, R., Bennett, K., Preece, T., & Phillipson, L. (2017). The development and testing of the dementia friendly communities environment assessment tool (DFC EAT). *International Psychogeriatrics*, 29(2), 303–311. https://doi.org/10.1017/S1041610216001678

Fleming, R., & Bowles, J. (1987). Units for the confused and disturbed elderly: Development, design, programming and evaluation. *Australian Journal on Ageing*, 6(4), 25–28. https://doi.org/10.1111/j.1741-6612.1987.tb01001.x

Fleming, R., & Purandare, N. (2010). Long-term care for people with dementia: Environmental design guidelines. *International Psychogeriatrics*, 22(7), 1084–1096. https://doi.org/10.1017/S1041610210000438

Fröst, P., & Warren, P. (2007). Virtual reality used in a collaborative architectural design process. Paper presented at the *2000 IEEE Conference on Information Visualization: An International Conference on Computer Visualization and Graphics*, London, UK. 568–573. https://doi.org/10.1109/IV.2000.859814

Grassini, S., & Laumann, K. (2020, November). Evaluating the use of virtual reality in work safety: A literature review. In *Proceedings of the 30th European safety and reliability conference and the 15th probabilistic safety assessment and management conference* (No. 3975).

Henry, G., Noel-Smith, J., Palmer, L., Quirke, M., & Wallace, K. (2021). *Environments for ageing and dementia design assessment tool.* University of Stirling.

Kerr, A. (2013). Body work in assisted conception: Exploring public and private settings. *Sociology of Health & Illness; Sociol Health Illn*, 35(3), 465–478. https://doi.org/10.1111/j.1467-9566.2012.01502.x

Kim, O., Pang, Y., & Kim, J. (2019). The effectiveness of virtual reality for people with mild cognitive impairment or dementia: A meta-analysis. *BMC Psychiatry*, 19(219), 1–10.

Kiuchi, D., Orura, A., Oishi, K. (2020) Japan: Experience of dementia design and education in Japan. In R. Fleming, J. Zeisel, & K. Bennett (Eds.), *World Alzheimer Report 2020: Design dignity dementia: Dementia-related design and the built environment volume I* (pp. 216–223). Alzheimer's Disease International. https://www.alz.co.uk/u/WorldAlzheimerReport2020Vol1.pdf

Kothgassner, O. D., Goreis, A., Kafka, J. X., Van Eickels, R. L., Plener, P. L., & Felnhofer, A. (2019). Virtual reality exposure therapy for posttraumatic stress disorder (PTSD): A meta-analysis. *European Journal of Psychotraumatology, 10*(1), 1654782. https://doi.org/10.1080/20008198.2019.1654782

Kvan, T. (2000). Collaborative design: What is it? *Automation in Construction, 9*(4), 409–415. https://doi.org/10.1016/S0926-5805(99)00025-4

Latham, M. (1994). *Constructing the team: Joint review of procurement and contractual arrangements in the United Kingdom construction industry.* HMSO. https://doi.org/10.1287/orsc.2013.0881

Manera, V., Chapoulie, E., Bourgeois, J., Guerchouche, R., David, R., Ondrej, J., Drettakis, G., & Robert, P. (2016). A feasibility study with image-based rendered virtual reality in patients with mild cognitive impairment and dementia. *PLoS One, 11*(3), e0151487. https://doi.org/10.1371/journal.pone.0151487

Marshall, M. (2001). The challenge of looking after people with dementia. *BMJ, 323*(7310), 410–411. https://doi.org/10.1136/bmj.323.7310.410

Maskey, M., Rodgers, J., Grahame, V., Glod, M., Honey, E., Kinnear, J., Labus, M., Milne, J., Minos, D., McConachie, H., & Parr, J. R. (2019). A randomised controlled feasibility trial of immersive virtual reality treatment with cognitive behaviour therapy for specific phobias in young people with autism spectrum disorder. *Journal of Autism and Developmental Disorders, 49*, 1912–1927. https://doi.org/ https://doi.org/10.1007/s10803-018-3861-x

Palmer, L., Wallace, K., & Hutchinson, L. (2021). *Architecture for dementia. Stirling Gold: 2008–2020.* University of Stirling.

Portman, M. E., Natapov, A., & Fisher-Gewirtzman, D. (2015). To go where no man has gone before: Virtual reality in architecture, landscape architecture and environmental planning. *Computers, Environment and Urban Systems, 54*, 376–384. https://doi.org/10.1016/j.compenvurbsys.2015.05.001

Rapoport, A. (1980). Cross-cultural aspects of environmental design. In A. Irman, R. Amos, & F. W. Joachim (Eds.), *Human behaviour and environment* (pp. 7–46). Springer. https://doi.org/10.1007/978-1-4899-0451-5_2

RIBA. (2020). *RIBA plan of work.* Retrieved May 30, 2023, from https://www.architecture.com/knowledge-and-resources/resources-landing-page/riba-plan-of-work

Riva, G., Riva, G., & Serino, S. (2021). *Virtual reality in the assessment, understanding and treatment of mental health disorders.* Multidisciplinary Digital Publishing Institute. https://doi.org/10.3390/books978-3-03943-776-4

Shapiro, J. (2008). Walking a mile in their patients' shoes: Empathy and othering in medical students' education. *Philosophy, Ethics, and Humanities in Medicine, 3*(1), 10. https://doi.org/10.1186/1747-5341-3-10

Shen, X. (2021). *Dementia eyes: Understanding dementia through augmented reality.* Master of Media Design. KeioUniversity https://koara.lib.keio.ac.jp/xoonips/modules/xoonips/detail.php?koara_id=KO40001001-00002021-0885

Shen, X., Pai, Y. S., Kiuchi, D., Bao, K., Aoki, T., Ando, R., Oishi, K., & Minami-zawa, K. (2021). Dementia eyes: Perceiving dementia with augmented reality. Paper presented at the *SIGGRAPH Asia 2021 XR (SA '21 XR)*, Tokyo, Japan (5) 1–2. https://doi.org/https://doi.org/10.1145/3478514.3487617

Sloane, P. D., Mitchell, C. M., Weisman, G., Zimmerman, S., Foley, K. M. L., Lynn, M., Calkins, M., Lawton, M. P., Teresi, J., Grant, L., Lindeman, D., & Montgomery, R. (2002). The therapeutic environment screening survey for nursing homes (TESS-NH): An observational instrument for assessing the physical environment of institutional settings for persons with dementia. *The Journals of Gerontology Series B: Psychological Sciences and Social Sciences*, 57(2), 69. https://doi.org/10.1093/geronb/57.2.s69

Succar, B. (2009). Building information modelling framework: A research and delivery foundation for industry stakeholders. *Automation in Construction*, 18(3), 357–375. https://doi.org/10.1016/j.autcon.2008.10.003

Tacken, M., Marcellini, F., Mollenkopf, H., Ruoppila, I., & Széman, Z. (2005). Use and acceptance of new technology by older people. Findings of the international MOBILATE survey: 'Enhancing mobility in later life'. *Gerontechnology*, 3(3), 126–137. https://journal.gerontechnology.org/archives/356-358-1-PB.pdf

The King's Fund. (2014). *Is your care home dementia friendly?: EHE environmental assessment tool* (2nd ed.) The King's Fund. https://www.kingsfund.org.uk/sites/default/files/field/field_pdf/is-your-care-home-dementia-friendly-ehe-tool-kingsfund-mar13.pdf

Zwoliński, G., Kamińska, D., Haamer, R. E., Pinto-Coelho, L., & Anbarjafari, G. (2023). Enhancing empathy through virtual reality: Developing a universal design training application for students. *Medycyna Pracy*, 74(3), 199–210. https://doi.org/10.13075/mp.5893.01407

6

Improving housing decisions for and with people with dementia

A co-design approach

Jodi Sturge and Louise Meijering

Introduction

Most people with dementia live at home. However, as physical and cognitive needs intensify, there is often a decision point for the person with dementia to move to suitable and supportive care environments (Moyle, 2019; Verbeek et al., 2012). Although modifying the home environment to support the well-being of persons with dementia is possible, there is often a lack of information available on how to adapt the home environment for dementia (Newton et al., 2021) and moving to a care environment is unavoidable. The critical decision is to move to a more supportive residential care environment. However, where and when to relocate depends on several factors related to the person with dementia, informal caregivers and resources (Verbeek et al., 2012). Ideally, housing decisions are made jointly with the person with dementia and caregivers. However, even in situations where the preferences of the person with dementia are clearly stated, their active contribution to the decision-making process decreases over time (Garvelink et al., 2019).

When it comes time to make housing decisions suitable for people with dementia, most people with dementia or caregivers are unaware of their options. To further complicate the decision-making process, people with dementia often fear losing independence and moving to unfamiliar institutional settings. Advanced care planning might help persons with dementia and caregivers to identify future needs more proactively (Read et al., 2017). Research suggests timely and honest communication helps mitigate the distress of deciding against the preferred option in advance care planning (Garvelink et al., 2019). Participatory research methods and collaborative research designs are becoming more common to strengthen the voice and participation of people at varying stages of dementia (Newton et al., 2021; Wang et al., 2019). Co-design is an iterative, interdisciplinary, participatory approach to design that situates individuals as experts who contribute their knowledge and skills to understand and solve the challenge or shared problem (Sanders & Stappers, 2014). Bringing people with dementia together with their caregivers and different disciplines for design can provide novel solutions to

DOI: 10.4324/9781003416241-9

problems (Ludden et al., 2019). Recognizing the expertise and knowledge of people with dementia through design research methods is considered a best practice for building self-esteem and dignity (Leorin et al., 2019; Rodgers et al., 2018).

The aim of this chapter is to describe a co-design research project which explored housing decision-making from the perspectives of the different stakeholders: people with dementia, informal caregivers, volunteers and professionals in dementia policy and care. The authors and an external design consulting firm (Koos Service Design) designed and implemented the transdisciplinary research project. Where there are no published design guidelines for designing with people with dementia (Wang et al., 2019), the firm and the designers were selected because they had experience doing design research with people with dementia. The co-design approach for this research was based on the Double Diamond Model (DDM) framework, which consists of four steps: Discover, Define, Develop and Deliver (West et al., 2018) (Figure 6.1). During the Discover the researchers gain a deeper understanding of the problem to solve. The Define step summarizes insights from the discovery step into a problem definition. Next, the Develop step encourages a variety of solutions to the defined problem. Finally, the Deliver step tests different solutions, rejecting the ones that do not work, and improving those with potential (West et al., 2018). The DDM is often used in co-design trajectories to sharpen the problem and identify potential solutions.

In line with the DDM, a five-day design sprint was used, a cost-effective method that consists of design activities to find solutions to a problem statement within a week (Knapp et al., 2016). This research activity occurred in Groningen, the Netherlands in October 2021. The research was part of the COORDINATES project, and ethical approval for the study was obtained from participating institutions. A cross-country comparison and reflection of the methods are described in other publications (Nordin et al., 2023; Sturge et al., 2021). Ethical board approval was obtained from the Ethics Research Committee, Faculty of Spatial Sciences, University of Groningen.

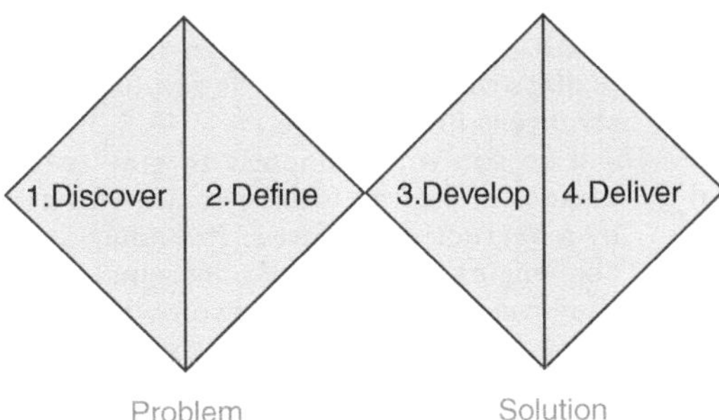

Figure 6.1 The double diamond design process.

The target group was older adults with memory problems or dementia who live at home and may face the possibility of moving to a care home. The authors contacted Odensehuis in Groningen, a stakeholder providing drop-in services to the target group. The service provider assisted with recruitment and provided office space for design research activities.

The co-design process and findings

Discovering and defining key themes

To gain a more profound and shared understanding of problems related to housing decisions for people with dementia, we provided the designers with background research and material related to the project, including feedback on the relevance of the topic offered by different stakeholders. Then, the authors and design researchers kicked off the five-day design sprint by setting expectations for the week. The authors and Koos Service Design coordinated interviews with people with dementia, informal caregivers, volunteers and professionals working in dementia care to understand and contextualize the 'problem' in the local context. The design researchers asked participants about their housing experiences and current living situation. They also discussed possible solutions to improve the living situation and choices about housing.

The conversations resulted in eight themes, which are summarized in Table 6.1.

Table 6.1 Key themes identified from interviews with participants

Key theme	Description
1 The essential role of informal caregivers for people with dementia	Participants described their experiences relying on a partner or family member. Having a partner to live with and to help with errands such as groceries brought comfort to people with dementia. However, when the partner disappears, whether through a divorce or death, the responsibility can shift to the children or professional home care. It can be challenging to have strangers in the house.
2 The physical and emotional challenges of providing informal care	For a person with dementia to stay at home as long as possible, often intensive informal care is provided by a partner or children. Providing such care can be challenging. For instance, informal caregivers feel that they cannot leave the person with dementia at home alone or that they do not have any time for themselves.

(Continued)

Table 6.1 (Continued)

Key theme	Description
3 A suboptimal healthcare system	Participants talked about the limited residential care options available, and when a space becomes available, it must be decided and arranged very quickly. This choice, however, does have financial implications. Participants talked about the cost of care. If you have a lot of money, there are choices and nice options such as care farms. Otherwise, arranging appropriate care and housing is very difficult.
4 Social contacts are vital for quality of life	People with dementia must maintain social contacts and have the option to meet up with people they know in close proximity. In addition, it is good if people continue to (learn and) display socially desirable behaviour. They 'practice' how it should be done and what makes them last longer in social contexts.
5 The move to a residential care environment is linked to decline in quality of life	It is difficult to get used to a new environment for some people with dementia. Participants stated they were unaware of how moving to a residential care environment worked well for an individual. They also talked about how moving to another environment in general, not even a care home, can result in the person with dementia deteriorating.
6 The need to move is often denied	People with dementia and their caregivers talked about making housing decisions 'someday', having the 'idea in their head' or that 'we are not that far yet, we are healthy.' However, others clearly stated that moving was not an option.
7 Orientating early and slowly getting used to a new living environment is helpful	Informal caregivers stated that they thought the conversation to move should happen once the diagnosis is made. They suggested that visiting the site before the actual move is helpful.
8 Living in a residential care environment: a compromise	Some participants described finding suitable housing that was small yet spacious and met their needs in the context of a senior home or assisted living. In contrast, people talked about the residential care environment negatively, describing it as a place where people with dementia lose their autonomy, and people want to continue to have a choice of what to eat or where to sleep.

Combining these experience themes with knowledge from previous research projects generated problem scenarios. Overall, the problem scenarios are characterized by unwanted residential disruptions and crises. When moving to a residential care environment, the usual daily ritual and social care can be disrupted, and people tend to deteriorate very quickly. As a result, residential care environments often have a negative association, making moving into such an environment a sensitive topic. Steps are usually only taken after crisis relief, and there is little opportunity to choose a suitable place. As a stakeholder explained, "(the decision) often happens after a crisis admission, for example, when the partner really cannot handle it anymore, or people set the house on fire and such." Additional insights included that talking about the subject can be accompanied by much emotion and may therefore be postponed. Then, delaying such a discussion typically means that it is postponed until a crisis happens. Crisis situations can include a critical incident such as a person with dementia becoming lost, injured by a fall or informal caregiver burnout. In such crises, a person with dementia may have to move urgently to a different living environment. As a result, often, no or little shared decisions or choices are made where the decision to move is based on available space, making a move to a new environment even more disruptive. Further, the care environments do not always include social care tailored to individual needs, like the services provided by groups. However, emerging practices ease the housing decision by creating environments specifically designed to be adapted to a person with dementia's progressive needs. One person with dementia told us about a housing project developer who advertised new housing units suitable for people with early-stage dementia.

Developing and delivering prototype solutions

The key themes generated in the discover and define phases were discussed between the authors and the design team to focus on the scope of the problem and potential solutions. This resulted in three opportunity statements, which guided the direction of the developed solutions (e.g., the prototypes) (Table 6.2).

Framing problems as opportunity statements allows for more positive discussions about housing types that may have negative associations. When people have a more positive image of a new housing option, it may be easier to discuss it and take action. This approach could positively affect the person with dementia and their informal caregivers, where the situation can be maintained (in a new home) for longer. Thus, the risk of a crisis of admission to a residential care environment can be reduced. People can be motivated to start orienting themselves on moving sooner and get used to moving slowly. If one begins to orientate on a possible move early, the person with memory problems can better map out requirements and wishes. By slowly getting used to moving, it is better to map out what suits someone and what does not. All this can ensure that the step to move becomes smaller. It can make the urgency more palpable among patients and caregivers so that the right choices are made sooner.

Table 6.2 Opportunity statements and their motivation

	Opportunity statement	Origin and motivation
1	How can we increase the urgency of moving earlier among the person with dementia and informal caregivers?	This statement comes from the opportunity area that slowly getting used to moving and starting early with orientation helps.
2	How can we make the future of housing a topic for discussion before people develop memory problems?	This statement comes from the opportunity area that highlights alternative housing options next to only the residential care environment with a negative image.
3	How can we make the transition from home to living in care more gradual for the person with dementia?	This statement comes from the opportunity area that helps people realize that moving positively affects their situation (or that of their loved ones).

With these opportunity statements in mind, the design team used a brainstorming session of out-of-the-box ideas and other best practices in healthcare with the authors to develop eight prototypes that would spark a conversation about dementia and moving. Prototypes included, (1) a documentary about living with dementia, (2) an information letter about housing options upon receiving a pension, (3) a board game, (4) a website that gives information about housing and care options, (5) a decision-making website, (6) a gradual move into a residential care environment with some visits before moving, (7) a buddy system and (8) a booklet containing the interests and background of the individual to be referred to a residential care environment.

The prototypes were presented to professionals who work in dementia care online in individual meetings (Figure 6.2). The professionals gave feedback on which prototype would be most relevant and promising to pursue further. Some prototypes, such as the documentary, were not chosen as ideal solutions due to cost. In contrast, other prototypes, like the website, were seen to already be in practice but needed to be better used and maintained with new information. The board game and the personal booklet were selected to develop. Both would require investment to fully develop, which was beyond the scope of our current project.

Feedback on the co-design method

Where our participatory co-design method is not standard in social sciences, we met with the professionals who tested the prototypes to get feedback on the process. The professionals described the research method as a new experience and fast-paced. One professional commented that the questions the designers asked seemed more random than systematically exploring the

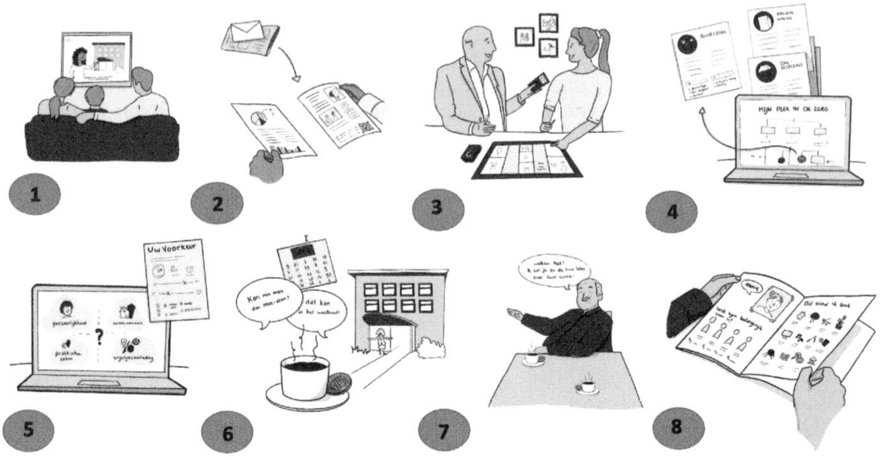

Figure 6.2 There were eight prototypes identified as possible solutions to improving housing decisions. Illustrated by Koos Service Design.

strengths and weaknesses of the prototypes. However, this approach was noted by the professionals to be beneficial, where they provided more spontaneous, rather than scripted, responses. Although the designers had some experience in dementia research, a professional mentioned that there were some parts of dementia care that the designers were not aware of, such as closed-door policies. Also, one professional recognized that the designers were from Amsterdam and unfamiliar with the dementia service structure of Groningen. However, it was noted that the designers were open to learning, and the professionals mentioned that they enjoyed working with young and enthusiastic people. After the session, the professionals said they later thought about the conversation and how it connected to their practice.

Conclusion

As people age, especially when living with chronic conditions like dementia, there are housing decisions to be made around location, levels of care, distance from familiar settings and family ties. When suitable housing is identified, this is not a guaranteed option where residential care environments are frequently fully occupied and have extensive waiting lists. As a result, the decision-making process is complex and does not always meet the wishes of the person with dementia. This problem is further complicated when the housing options obtained in a crisis are based solely on emergency availability, not a preferred choice by the person with dementia or their family members.

Using a co-design approach, we explored solutions that better facilitate preliminary conversations about housing decisions for people with dementia.

This chapter summarizes the results from a co-design project that provided insightful perspectives from various disciplines and lived experience levels. Specifically, we wanted to identify prototypes that could increase the interest, urgency, and choice to facilitate a person-centred and more gradual transition to a residential care environment. This type of participatory research approach aligns with a transdisciplinary mode which is becoming more common to identify problems to complex social issues (Population Europe, 2022). The benefit of a co-design approach, as described by Sanders and Stappers (2014), is to combine the expertise of the authors, the creativity of the designers and engaging stakeholders not trained in the method, which results in identifying prototype solutions to a problem. Eight prototypes were identified as possible conversation starters to support housing decisions for people with dementia, which three professionals tested. Ideally, more stakeholders would have tested these prototypes, including people with dementia, informal care providers or physicians and architects. Also, as noted by Wang et al. (2019), the short duration of five days as well as the small sample size make it difficult to generalize the findings. Additionally, only the voices of people with dementia accessing services at Odensehuis were explored, noting the voices of people not accessing services were not considered. Also, the prototypes were not tested with people with dementia. It was decided not to have people with dementia participate in the prototype testing based on cautionary statements made by Lindsay et al. (2012), who suggest that people with dementia can have challenges recalling previous experiences or imagining future scenarios. However, for future co-design, we would like people with dementia to decide whether they want to participate in that design phase or not. A more immersive design ethnography inclusive of a more diverse sample of participants over a more extended period would produce more detailed and rigorous findings. Although the design research team had experience with design and dementia research and was provided with a research overview by the authors, the nuances related to dementia care policies and the local service context were missing. For future studies in dementia care, the design researchers would ideally be from the region and have more policy experience. Also, to ensure the viability of the development of the prototype, collaborations with a game and activity developer like Relish (relish-life.com) would support the likelihood of a prototype being created, evaluated and made available for people with dementia.

Despite the limited sample size and time frame, co-design provided several insights into the problem and solutions related to housing decisions for people with dementia living in Groningen. For people with dementia, informal caregivers and stakeholders were engaged in the process. Further, through co-design, we could improve other dementia care processes by understanding how individuals experience navigating the healthcare system. This level of understanding would provide opportunities to explore improving policy, process or systems, not necessarily related to designing a product or technology.

In-depth box

- This co-design research project explored housing decision-making from the perspectives of the different stakeholders, including people with dementia, informal caregivers, volunteers and professionals in dementia policy and care.
- Through the design process, opportunity statements were combined with other research knowledge to create problem scenarios.
- Two prototypes (a board game and a personal booklet) were chosen as suitable solutions to improve communication and choice related to housing decisions for and with people with dementia.
- Developing these protypes could improve housing decision-making for people with dementia by initiating conversations and choices based on preferences around location, levels of care, distance from familiar settings or family ties.

Acknowledgements

We would like to thank Koos Service Design for their support with this project and coordinating the data collection. Also, we would like to acknowledge the commitment and energy of the staff and volunteers from Odensehuis in Groningen.

This publication is a part of the COORDINATEs study (project number: 9003037412) which is funded by the Joint Programming Initiative More Years, Better Lives, represented by ZonMw in the Netherlands.

References

Garvelink, M. M., Groen-van de Ven, L., Smits, C., Franken, R., Dassen-Vernooij, M., & Légaré, F. (2019). Shared decision making about housing transitions for persons with dementia: a four-case care network perspective. *The Gerontologist*, *59*(5), 822–834.

Knapp, J., Zeratsky, J., & Kowitz, B. (2016). *Sprint: How to solve big problems and test new ideas in just five days*. Simon and Schuster.

Leorin, C., Stella, E., Nugent, C., Cleland, I., & Paggetti, C. (2019). The value of including people with dementia in the co-design of personalized eHealth technologies. *Dementia and geriatric cognitive disorders*, *47*(3), 164–175.

Lindsay, S., Brittain, K., Jackson, D., Ladha, C., Ladha, K., & Olivier, P. (2012). Empathy, participatory design and people with dementia. In *Proceedings of the SIGCHI conference on Human factors in computing systems* (pp. 521–530).

Ludden, G. D., van Rompay, T. J., Niedderer, K., & Tournier, I. (2019). Environmental design for dementia care-towards more meaningful experiences through design. *Maturitas*, *128*, 10–16.

Moyle, W. (2019). The promise of technology in the future of dementia care. *Nature Reviews Neurology*, *15*(6), 353–359.

Newton, R., Adams, S., Keady, J., & Tsekleves, E. (2021). Exploring the contribution of housing adaptations in supporting everyday life for people with dementia: a scoping review. *Ageing & Society*, *43*(8), 1833–1859.

Nordin, S., Sturge, J., Meijering, L., & Elf, M. (2023). A 5-day codesign sprint to improve housing decisions of older adults: lessons learned from Sweden and the Netherlands. *International Journal of Social Research Methodology*, 1–13. https://doi.org/10.1080/13645579.2023.2247290

Population Europe (2022). *Transdisciplinarity: a research mode for real world problems*, 49. https://population-europe.eu/research/discussion-papers/transdisciplinarity

Read, S. T., Toye, C., & Wynaden, D. (2017). Experiences and expectations of living with dementia: a qualitative study. *Collegian*, *24*(5), 427–432.

Rodgers, P. A. (2018). Co-designing with people living with dementia. *CoDesign*, *14*(3), 188–202.

Sanders, E. B. N., & Stappers, P. J. (2014). Probes, toolkits and prototypes: three approaches to making in codesigning. *CoDesign*, *10*(1), 5–14.

Sturge, J., Meijering, L., Jones, C. A., Garvelink, M., Caron, D., Nordin, S., ... & Légaré, F. (2021). Technology to improve autonomy and inform housing decisions for older adults with memory problems who live at home in Canada, Sweden, and the Netherlands: protocol for a multipronged mixed methods study. *JMIR Research Protocols*, *10*(1), e19244.

Verbeek, H., Meyer, G., Leino-Kilpi, H., Zabalegui, A., Hallberg, I. R., Saks, K., ... & RightTimePlaceCare Consortium. (2012). A European study investigating patterns of transition from home care towards institutional dementia care: the protocol of a RightTimePlaceCare study. *BMC Public Health*, *12*, 1–10.

Wang, G., Marradi, C., Albayrak, A., & van der Cammen, T. J. (2019). Co-designing with people with dementia: a scoping review of involving people with dementia in design research. *Maturitas*, *127*, 55–63.

West, J., Fusari, G., Raby, E., Alwani, R., Meldaikyte, G., Wojdecka, A., & Matthews, E. (2018). Developing the double diamond process for implementation. In: D. Barron & K. Seemann, (eds.) *Design4Health, Melbourne. Proceedings of the fourth international conference on Design4Health 2017*, 4–7 December 2017, Melbourne, Victoria, Australia. Sheffield Hallam University and Swinburne University of Technology, pp. 310–312. ISBN 978-0-6480892-1-6.

Dementia friendly neighbourhoods

How can public organizations, transport systems and spaces be made more dementia friendly? Findings from participatory health research and architecture

*Verena C. Tatzer, Barbara Pichler,
Elisabeth Reitinger, Gesine Marquardt
and Katharina Heimerl*

Why public organizations have to become dementia-sensitive and more inclusive

People with dementia and their caregivers often experience restrictions in social participation (Thalén et al., 2022). Communities and public organizations need to adapt their services to the needs of older people and people living with cognitive disorders. Libraries and museums are buildings that should be as accessible as possible since they serve many purposes in the community. For people with dementia, libraries and museums can be spaces to spend time, retrieve information, interact with others, but also to find respite in a busy urban area. Other public buildings, such as town-hall citizens' information service offices may not be leisure spaces. Nevertheless, they still need to be easily accessible for people with dementia – regardless of whether they visit to deal with official matters or if they need a space for respite during their day. Public transport systems are an essential component to ensure that people with dementia can continue to participate in their community and get around, especially after ceasing to drive themselves.

Yet there is surprisingly little to be found in literature regarding dementia-friendly environmental design to improve public organizations and spaces for people with cognitive impairment. Research on accessibility in public or semi-public spaces, such as grocery stores (Brorsson et al., 2020) or neighborhoods (Ward et al., 2018) from the perspective of people with dementia, is still woefully scarce and there is a lack of studies examining how the spatial environment can support people with dementia in their leisure activities (Woodbridge et al., 2018).

This chapter presents lessons learned from participatory projects in Austria that focused on the physical and social environment and people with

DOI: 10.4324/9781003416241-11

dementia: "The Dementia-friendly Library Wiener Neustadt" that included a library, a museum and a town-hall citizens' information service (Heimerl et al., submitted; Pichler et al., 2023; Tatzer et al., 2022a, 2022b, in press) as well as projects that focused on public transport and mobility (Knoll et al., 2018; Pichler et al., 2019; Reitinger et al., 2018 a,b). Together with the principles of dementia-friendly architecture (Büter & Marquardt, 2021), we aim to provide some insight into how public institutions and spaces can be transformed into more inclusive places.

The methods used in the projects were diverse: ranging from focus groups (Heimerl et al., submitted) to walking interviews (Pichler et al., 2023; Reitinger et al., 2018) to workshops with photos and online surveys (Tatzer et al., 2022a). The common element of the projects was the participation of people with dementia and their caregivers: as members of the steering committee, as research participants, but also as advocates and referees. Participatory research is about exploring and influencing social reality in partnership (von Unger, 2012). Thus, the focus is on a dual objective: on the one hand, to gain scientific knowledge and, on the other hand, to change reality and intervene in social systems as part of the process of knowledge acquisition.

Orientation and outdoor mobility of people with dementia

Many studies highlight the important role of neighborhood and their environment for daily outdoor activity (Clarke et al., 2015; Keady et al., 2012; Mitchell & Burton, 2006; Ward et al., 2018; Woodbridge et al., 2018). Brorsson et al. (2011) found that even small changes in public space, for example, a repainted house, influenced their orientation and perceived accessibility. Here we present the results of a study on the mobility of people with dementia (Knoll et al., 2018; Pichler et al., 2019; Reitinger et al., 2018). The aim of this study was to gather knowledge for public transport planners, urban planners and caregivers on how best to support people with dementia to move around independently.

Based on a qualitative research approach, narrative interviews, guided neighborhood walks and public transport were used with people with mild dementia to explore their everyday experiences and strategies for getting around outdoors. A deeper understanding of typical behavioral patterns in 'being on the move' emerged from the analysis of the narrative interviews. The qualitative data were analyzed with the "Documentary method" by Bohnsack (2014) that resulted in a typology of two different ways of mobility and orientation. One characterization can be called "social orientation" (type one), the other "individual orientation" (type two) (Pichler et al., 2019).

In principle, type one is characterized by a social and communicative attitude. Everyday activities, as well as mobility in public space and on public transport, can be interpreted as socially embedded. Other people are involved in actions and are important motivators for this type 1. Talking to each other seems quite 'natural' and everybody seems to be a potential dialogue partner. With regard to outdoor mobility, the main orientation strategy for persons of type one – especially in situations when the person cannot find the way – is to ask other people.

The main characteristic of type two on the other hand is that the person themselves is at the center of their action. This means that persons of this type organize themselves and act in a planned way both in their everyday activities and in their use of transport. When faced with challenges and problems, these persons try to solve them on their own. This requires a high degree of self-discipline and includes personal training. Getting around and using public transport is seen as an important factor of keeping fit – both physically and mentally. Memory training and reading are seen as good ways to combat memory loss. They prefer planning and other strategies before asking someone for help. Maps are studied and new routes are practiced in advance. Some narratives also show that such people are willing to take the risk of getting lost because they want to travel independently.

People need different things depending on their type, according to our findings. The first type 'social orientation', which is described as social and communicative, requires people to ask questions directly to find their way. Traveling in a metropolitan area also means using public transport. It is therefore important that the public transport operator has information points and staff available to answer questions. The restructuring of ticket machines and digital information is very problematic for this type. These results show the importance of interpersonal contacts in public spaces. Therefore, if a society wants to be dementia-friendly, everyone needs to be informed about dementia. It is particularly important to know how to communicate appropriately in everyday situations and in situations where the person needs help. These findings highlight the importance of dementia-friendly initiatives and campaigns. If people with dementia of this type cannot go out alone, it is important to have the opportunity to go for walks or excursions together and to have an assistant.

The second type, people with an "individual orientation", need a different kind of support. Their intuitive strategy is not to ask anyone, but to find their way around first. They therefore need a dementia-sensitive architecture and spatial orientation markers. Such markers can be a prominent building such as a church or a particular shop. They need timetables and orientation maps which are easy to read and understand as well as easy to use technical aids.

These types do not appear only with the diagnosis of dementia, but build up biographically. The importance of these strategies is specific to people with dementia. However, they are even more important for people with disorientation in order to be able to orient themselves both indoors and outdoors.

Dementia-sensitive architecture

Dementia-sensitive communities support the idea of people with dementia participating in public life. In several studies, facilitators and barriers to community engagement for people with dementia have been identified. They are manifold, but with regards to architectural design, key aspects such as worrying about getting lost, getting confused by street layouts or unclear signs, feeling overwhelmed in crowded situations, and embarrassment about the symptoms of dementia have emerged (Shannon et al., 2019).

However, dementia-friendly design of public buildings and spaces is still fairly uncommon. Back in 2003, the Iris Murdoch Building of the Dementia Services Development Centre at the University of Stirling was opened and it still serves as a showcase of dementia-sensitive design principles applied to a public building (McCabe & Sim, 2006). In the view of the authors, it is rather disappointing to realize that the potential of public buildings as facilitators to community engagement for people with dementia has not been fully understood and appreciated yet. In wayfinding studies, public buildings have been identified as important landmarks for orientation, and the importance of implementing environmental interventions to optimize dementia-sensitive spaces has been addressed (Kuliga et al., 2021).

Principles of dementia-sensitive architecture

Research on architectural design that supports the health and wellbeing of people with dementia has already been conducted for more than forty years. The environments which have been investigated are rather limited, including either health care institutions (such as nursing homes, long-term care and adult day care settings and hospitals) or housing (such as shared dwellings, assisted living and individual homes). However, the literature coherently concludes that dementia-sensitive architecture is helpful for the individuals living with dementia and their caregivers (Fleming et al., 2020).

Building on these findings, Büter and Marquardt (2021) identified 10 principles of dementia-sensitive architecture. They include guidance on 1. *the floor plan structure, 2. floor space requirements, 3. safety, 4. orientation, 5. guidance and orientation systems, 6. lighting, 7. colors and contrasts, 8. atmosphere, 9. activation concepts* and 10. *stimulus densities.* As with most of the literature in this field, these principles pertain mainly to the field of health-care design. Nevertheless, regarding the underlying relationship between the needs of people with dementia and the built environment, it becomes evident that these principles are generalizable and can be applied to the architectural design of public buildings, ultimately addressing the main physical barriers to community engagement for people with dementia.

Implementation in public buildings

To implement dementia-sensitive design in public buildings, it is feasible to apply the postulated design principles.

1 <u>Floorplan structure:</u> Simple, clearly defined building structures and room layouts help people with dementia to find their way around. Spatial anchor points are key elements to be included. They are highly recognizable places that are meaningful for the users of the building. For example, this could be the seating area opposite an information desk in the foyer, to allow for rest and observation of the goings-on in the building.
2 <u>Floor space requirements:</u> Dementia is associated with advancing age, as well as declining stamina and physical fitness. As a result, many people with dementia rely on mobility aids such as walking frames or wheelchairs. Movement areas and corridors must therefore be generous in size to allow visitors to move around safely.
3 <u>Safety:</u> Regulations for barrier-free, accessible design ensure the safety of people with dementia moving about in a public building. Accommodating for visual loss by using intense color contrasts or additionally providing audible information is necessary as well. Furthermore, hazards can be reduced by implementing visual barriers, e.g., camouflaging doors or items with an inconspicuous appearance.
4 <u>Orientation:</u> Design that supports wayfinding not only facilitates the direct navigation of those with dementia to their intended destination in the building, it can also help with their temporal orientation and support situational comprehension of their own presence in the environment. This helps understanding how others expect them to behave in this space (e.g., being quiet in the reading room of a library) and might reduce possible occasions for embarrassment due to the symptoms of dementia.
5 <u>Guidance and orientation systems:</u> They are helpful for everyone who is a new or infrequent user of a public building. However, while multiple methods of signaling and addressing different senses to convey information is necessary to support the orientation and wayfinding abilities of those with dementia, excess information can easily lead to sensory overload. Therefore, it is important to focus on the essentials and omit non-vital information, such as decorative elements.
6 <u>Lighting:</u> Older adults need indoor lighting that is bright, even and glare-free. This enables them to see and perceive a room as a whole. Light is not only essential for vision, but also for communication, as it allows people with hearing problems to better see the accompanying facial expressions and gestures of the speaker. Finally, lighting can be used for the support of orientation and wayfinding, as specific areas and objects can be emphasized and enhanced with special lighting.

7 <u>Colors and contrasts:</u> Age-related visual impairments can at least partially be compensated for through the careful use of colors and contrasts. In floor coverings, strong contrasts, color changes or patterns should be avoided as they can be interpreted as obstacles and impair peoples' gait, even leading to falls. Most importantly, it should be noted that there is no scientific evidence on how certain colors affect individuals living with dementia.

8 <u>Atmosphere:</u> People with dementia may perceive a visit to an unfamiliar public building as daunting. It is important to make them feel welcome and appreciated, which is achieved by friendly and aesthetically pleasing interior design, a spatial structure that induces communication, social interaction, and participation. Creating an ambience that gives people with dementia security and orientation is a prerequisite.

9 <u>Activation concepts:</u> Visits to public buildings can be very helpful to prevent functional and cognitive decline. Activities can include participation in events tailored to the needs of people with dementia, but also spontaneous interaction with other people encountered in the public spaces.

10 <u>Stimulus densities:</u> Dementia limits the ability to filter environmental impressions, process them correctly, interpret them meaningfully and respond appropriately. Accordingly, environmental stimuli can quickly become too much for individuals living with dementia. Therefore, it is necessary to balance stimulation and calm. Environmental information needs to be used sparingly and attention span of those with dementia should be directed specifically at the relevant spaces. This includes restricting signage to the most important information, limiting decoration, minimizing acoustic stimuli and avoiding frequent changes in color and material.

Examples of implementation in public organizations

The project "The dementia friendly library Wiener Neustadt" aimed to foster social participation of people with dementia and their caregivers as well as to contribute to de-stigmatization and to increase health literacy in the general public. The needs assessment in the participatory health research project included focus groups with caregivers of people with dementia and walking interviews with caregivers and people living with dementia.

Workshops on topics such as communication, architectural and environmental design issues and health literacy were developed based on the identified needs and conducted with staff from the regional museum, public library and town-hall citizens' information service. All interventions were developed in collaboration with the local Alzheimer Austria self-help group including an activist living with cognitive impairment. The workshop on dementia-sensitive architecture and design was particularly important because its principles were considered easy to understand and some of the improvements suggested which had been identified in the workshop using photos and walking interviews could then be easily implemented. Examples of environmental changes included improved signage, the installation of clocks and the purchase of furniture and additional seating in the library and museum (Tatzer et al., 2022). Figure 7.1 shows an area that is designed to be seen from the information point where a librarian sits – so that a person living with dementia can rest safely and enjoy newspapers while, e.g., a relative is looking for information in the library. By its design and location, this area is designated to serve as a spatial anchor point.

Suggestions developed by occupational therapy students to improve the guidance systems (Depisch, 2022) and signage in the town-hall citizens' information service (Altenburger, 2023) were presented to officials during the projects and will be implemented peu à peu as and when renovations are needed.

The changes in the environment resulted in "quick wins" that were visible and sustainable (Zepke & Finsterwald, 2022). A symbol of the museum's readiness to change was the replacement of a former white toilet seat with a dark blue one (following the principle of contrasting colors and dementia-sensitive design), see Figure 7.2.

All the heads of the organizations involved reported back that learning about dementia-friendly architecture and design led to an increased awareness of the diversity of needs of other groups, such as people with physical disabilities, mobility issues, but also sensory issues, such as hearing or visual impairments. It is therefore helpful to link the term "dementia-friendly" with broader approaches under a term such as inclusion (Tatzer et al., 2022; Zepke & Finsterwald, 2022).

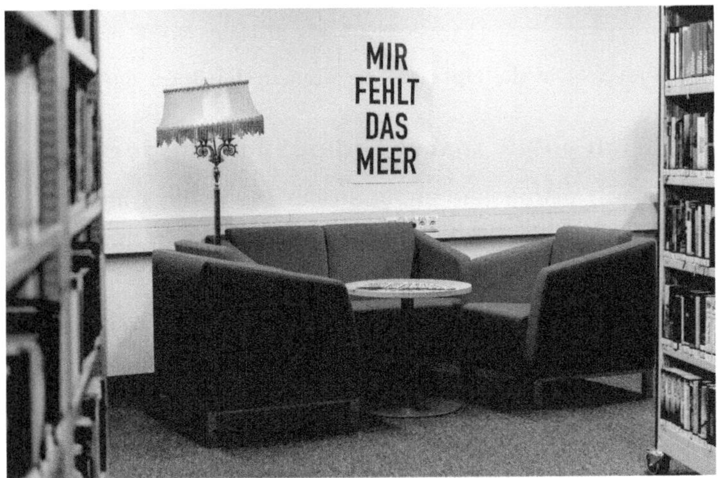

Figure 7.1 Seating area and spatial anchor point in sight of the librarian @AndreaLenc.

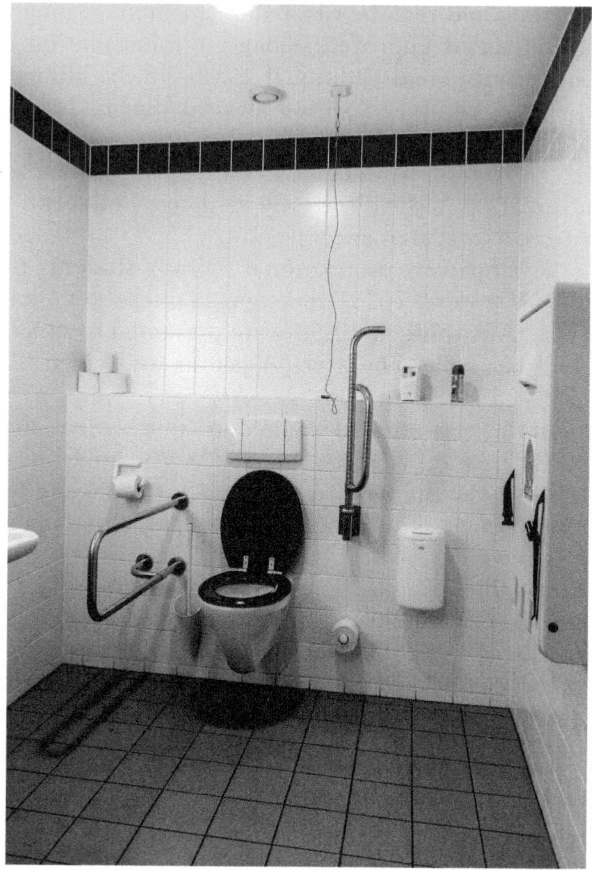

Figure 7.2 Toilet seat in the Museum St. Peter an der Sperr @AndreaLenc.

Examples from public spaces and public transport

Dementia-friendly planning in public spaces and public transport faces similar challenges to dementia-sensitive architecture. A crucial question that emerged during our research process in two different projects ("dementia on the move" and "people with dementia in public transport" (Knoll et al., 2018; Pichler et al., 2019; Reitinger et al., 2018a, 2018b) was: What does "dementia-friendly" planning in public spaces and public transport actually mean?

The main finding from the different methodological approaches was that the mobility of people with dementia in public spaces and on public transport is not only limited by cognitive impairments, but also to a large extent by physical impairments. Particularly with the focus on mobility, dementia appears to be an aspect of multimorbidity in old age. Dementia-related impairments in old age often occur in combination with limited physical mobility and declining sensory abilities.

This leads to the conclusion that dementia-friendly planning must build on the previously identified age-friendly and barrier-free planning of public spaces and public transport and also consider the cognitive dimension. One participant spoke of an "orientation-friendly environment" that helps people with dementia to find their way around.

Important aspects to consider are:

- The quality of open spaces: a quiet place without any traffic where people with dementia can enjoy greenery and rest comfortably on a bench. It is therefore essential to provide seating, which is both ample and well-designed.
- The quality of the flooring: barrier-free use of public spaces requires a level and transition-free ground floor with even sidewalks so that walking aids can be easily used.
- Public toilets are essential to support the mobility of people with dementia in public spaces.

As demonstrated above, the two dimensions of the physical and technical environment, on the one hand, and the social environment, on the other, need to be addressed in the process of dementia-friendly planning for public spaces and public transport.

Lessons learned and recommendations

In summarizing the challenges and recommendations, we want to focus on some lessons learned.

Ensuring the participation of people with dementia and their caregivers/next of kin

A key learning from the projects presented is the value of involving people with dementia in the research design and project architecture. Including people with dementia in the steering committee and ensuring participation was an essential factor in its success. Resources have to be budgeted to support the preparation of steering committee meetings, but also to support people with more advanced dementia while their caregivers participate in a focus group.

In the projects presented, the person with cognitive impairment in the steering group was supported by an assistant. The research team made sure that all steps were planned well in advance and that roles and tasks were clearly communicated during the workshops. This direct involvement not only leads to more sustainable outcomes. It also has the potential to empower people with dementia and their caregivers. Involvement reactivated social roles and identities that have been submerged, such as being a member of the library and a reader or opportunities for participation, such as visiting the museum and pursuing one's own interests despite being a caregiver (Pichler et al., 2023). A major limitation is involving more diverse people with dementia, as the representatives we were able to reach were mainly from educated backgrounds, mostly female and white. When considering what kind of support people with dementia need to get around and to participate for as long as possible, it is important to consider aspects of diversity and inequality. Gender, the socio-economic situation, migration background and other diversity categories have a strong influence on living situation and possible access to support systems (Roes et al. 2022).

Involving the social environment and caregivers

We want to stress the recommendation to include the social environment of people with dementia, as people with dementia often do things together with family members or friends, especially if they are afraid of getting lost or have additional health and mobility problems. In particular, in the projects the authors conducted concerning mobility in public spaces and public transport, it became clear that people with dementia may at some point need companions to help them find their way. We recommend the separate treatment of the two perspectives, that of the person with cognitive impairment and that of the caregiver, family or friend. In public institutions it is key to educate, train and involve staff to develop sustainable changes.

Human needs as a starting point for architecture and design

It is important to note that complying with the principles of dementia-sensitive architecture does not lead to a "lesser" design or restrict the architects' creativity. Many design projects showed that the principles of dementia-sensitive architecture can be implemented in an aesthetically pleasing way. Moreover, by considering human needs as the focus of all design measures, dementia-friendly architecture promotes the development of a holistic, inclusive design approach and creates a more accessible built environment (Kirch & Marquardt, 2021). As such, dementia-sensitive design, in the view of the authors, is a driver for human-centered design, leading to more inclusive environments.

Conclusion

The physical environment and its development in organizations is particularly fruitful in interdisciplinary and participatory research projects with (older) people with dementia because it offers concrete conditions and opportunities for participation to improve aspects of accessibility, but also symbolic meanings that can anchor identity and offer potential for social roles and participation. Our results show that the dimensions of the physical (and technical) environment, on the one hand, and the social environment, on the other hand, need to be considered in the process of dementia-friendly planning in public spaces and public transport. A transactional perspective that considers these dimensions together with the dimension of the activities which will be carried out in the environment can be helpful in developing dementia-friendly places. The concreteness of everyday life as manifested in the physical environment can contribute to a shared public space that offers potential for citizens to participate and live in, as well as a place for creating meaning and changing discourses and images of what it means to live as an aging person with cognitive impairment.

In-depth box

- Using participatory research including people with dementia and their carers to develop an inclusive physical environment is recommended.
- The transaction of both the physical and social environments as well as factors associated with the person and the activities done need to be addressed in an organization to become more inclusive.
- Methods like walking interviews that capture the transaction of the persons, activities and environment in the situation were successful in creating sustainable changes.

Acknowledgements

The project "The Dementia-friendly Library Wiener Neustadt" was funded by the Austrian public health institute (Fonds Gesundes Österreich) with the project number 3084. The project "Dementia on the move" was funded by the Austrian Research Promotion Agency (FFG), project number 855001 and the project "People with dementia in public transport" was funded by the "Federal Ministry of Social Affairs, Health, Care and Consumer Protection"

References

Altenburger, S. V. (2023). *Die demenzsensible, barrierefreie Bürgerservicestelle. Demenzfreundliche Beschilderung nach universellem Design* [The dementia-sensitive, barrier-free Citizen Information Service Point. Dementia-friendly signage and universal design]. [Bachelor's thesis, University of Applied Sciences Wiener Neustadt]. Wiener Neustadt.

Bohnsack, R. (2014). Documentary Method. In U. Flick (Ed.), *The SAGE handbook of qualitative data analysis* (pp. 217–233). London: Sage.

Brorsson, A., Öhman, A., Lundberg, S., Cutchin, M. P., & Nygård, L. (2020). How accessible are grocery shops for people with dementia? A qualitative study using photo documentation and focus group interviews. *Dementia (London)*, *19*(6), 1872–1888. https://doi.org/10.1177/1471301218808591

Brorsson, A., Ohman, A., Lundberg, S., & Nygard, L. (2011). Accessibility in public space as perceived by people with Alzheimer's disease. *Dementia*, *10*(4), 587–602. https://doi.org/10.1177/1471301211415314

Büter, K., & Marquardt, G. (2021). *Dementia-friendly hospital buildings. Construction and Design Manual*. DOM Publishing.

Clarke, P. J., Weuve, J., Barnes, L., Evans, D. A., & Mendes de Leon, C. F. (2015). Cognitive decline and the neighborhood environment. *Annals of Epidemiology*, *25*(11), 849–854. https://doi.org/10.1016/j.annepidem.2015.07.001

Depisch, C. (2022). *Bürgerservicestelle Wiener Neustadt - Anregungen und Empfehlungen zur demenzfreundlichen Gestaltung und Förderung der Orientierung* [Town Hall Information Service - Suggestions and Recommendations for a dementia friendly design to improve orientation]. [Bachelor's thesis, University of Applied Sciences Wiener Neustadt]. Wiener Neustadt. www.fhwn.ac.at/dembib

Fleming, R., Zeisel, J., & Bennett, K. (2020). *World Alzheimer Report 2020: Design Dignity Dementia: dementia-related design and the built environment. Volume 1.* https://www.alzint.org/u/WorldAlzheimerReport2020Vol1.pdf

Heimerl, K., Pichler, B., Plunger, P., & Tatzer, V. C. (submitted). Experiences with people with dementia in public community organizations – challenges in becoming dementia-friendly

Keady, J., Campbell, S., Barnes, H., Ward, R., Li, X., Swarbrick, C., … Elvish, R. (2012). Neighbourhoods and dementia in the health and social care context: A realist review of the literature and implications for UK policy development. *Reviews in Clinical Gerontology*, *22*(2), 150–163. https://doi.org/10.1017/S0959259811000268

Kirch, J., & Marquardt, G. (2021). Towards human-centered general hospitals: The potential of dementia-friendly design. *Architectural Science Review*, 1–9. https://doi.org/10.1080/00038628.2021.1933889

Knoll, B., Hofleitner, B., Reitinger, E., Pichler, B., & Egger, B. (2018). Dementia on the move: Preliminary results based on a participative qualitative research project focusing on the daily mobility patterns of people with dementia. *Collection of Open Conferences in Research Transport*. https://doi.org/10.5281/zenodo.1456409

Kuliga, S., Berwig, M., & Roes, M. (2021). Wayfinding in people with Alzheimer's disease: Perspective taking and architectural cognition—A vision paper on future dementia care research opportunities. *Sustainability*, *13*(3), 1084. https://www.mdpi.com/2071-1050/13/3/1084

McCabe, L., & Sim, D. (2006). Working in a 'dementia-friendly' office: Stirling University's Iris Murdoch Building. *Design Studies*, *27*(5), 615–632.

Mitchell, L., & Burton, E. (2006). Neighbourhoods for life: Designing dementia-friendly outdoor environments. *Quality in Ageing and Older Adults*, *7*(1), 26–33. https://doi.org/10.1108/14717794200600005

Pichler, B., Heimerl, K., & Tatzer, V. C. (2023). Creating a library, museum and citizen service centre for people with dementia. A project on participation and learning through transdisciplinary and interdisciplinary networking in Wiener

Neustadt [Bibliothek, Museum und Bürgerservicestelle für Menschen mit Demenz gestalten. Ein Projekt zu Partizipation und Lernen durch trans- und interdisziplinäre Vernetzung in Wiener Neustadt]. *Erwachsenenbildung.at. Das Fachmedium für Forschung, Praxis und Diskurs*, 48. https://erwachsenenbildung.at/magazin/23-48/12-bibliothek-museum-und-buergerservicestelle-fuer-menschen-mit-demenz-gestalten-pichler-heimerl-tatzer.pdf

Pichler, B., Hofleitner, B., Knoll, B., Renkin, A., Egger, B., & Reitinger, E. (2019). Forschungsbericht "Gut unterwegs mit Demenz in der Stadt? Spannungsfelder & Mobilitätsmuster im öffentlichen Raum" (Grundlagenstudie) [Getting around well in the city with dementia? Tensions and patterns of mobility in public space]. https://unterwegs-mit-demenz.at/wp-content/uploads/2019/10/Grundlagenstudie.pdf

Reitinger, E., Egger, B., Heimerl, K., Knoll, B., & Hellmer, S. (2018a) (BMASGK). *Menschen mit Demenz im öffentlichen Verkehr. Handlungsempfehlungen für Mitarbeiterinnen und Mitarbeiter in Verkehrsunternehmen* [People with dementia and public transport. Recomendations for staff in transport companies]. https://broschuerenservice.sozialministerium.at/Home/Download?publicationId=69&attachmentName=Menschen_mit_Demenz_im_%C3%B6ffentlichen_Verkehr_2018_pdfUA.pdf

Reitinger, E., Pichler, B., Egger, B., Knoll, B., Hofleitner, B., Plunger, P., Dressel, G., & Heimerl, K. (2018b). Research with people with Dementia—Ethical reflections on qualitative research praxis on mobility in public space. *Forum Qualitative Sozialforschung/Forum: Qualitative Social*, 19(3). https://doi.org/10.17169/fqs-19.3.3152

Roes, M., Laporte Uribe, F., Peters-Nehrenheim, V., Smits, C., Johannessen, A., Charlesworth, G., Parveen, S., Mueller, N., Hedd Jones, C., Thyrian, R., Monsees, J., & Tezcan-Güntekin, H. (2022). Intersectionality and its relevance for research in dementia care of people with a migration background. *Zeitschrift für Gerontologie und Geriatrie*, 55(4), 287–291. https://doi.org/10.1007/s00391-022-02058-y

Shannon, K., Bail, K., & Neville, S. (2019). Dementia-friendly community initiatives: An integrative review. *Journal of Clinical Nursing*, 28(11–12), 2035–2045. https://doi.org/10.1111/jocn.14746

Tatzer, V. C., Pichler, B., & Heimerl, K. (2022a). *"Eine Bibliothek für Alle - die demenzfreundliche Bibliothek Wiener Neustadt" - Endbericht zur Verbreitung der Projekterfahrungen und Ergebnisse* [A library for all - the dementia-friendly library Wiener Neustadt - Project Report for disseminating Findings and Experiences.]. u. report. https://fgoe.org/sites/fgoe.org/files/project-attachments/DemBib_Endbericht_27%2012%202022.pdf

Tatzer, V. C., Pichler, B., Plunger, P., Ullmer, R., & Heimerl, K. (2022b). *Gut leben mit Demenz in der Gemeinde. Bibliothek, Museum, Bürgerservicestelle für ALLE. Projekthandbuch* [Living well with dementia in the community. Library, Museum, Citizen Information Point for ALL. Project handbook] https://dzm8y13tmaxsv.cloudfront.net/wiener_neustadt/DemBib-Projekthandbuch_2022.pdf

Tatzer, V. C., Pichler, B., Reitinger, E., Plunger, P., & Heimerl, K. (in press). Demenzfreundliche Organisationen durch partizipative Forschung. Partizipation als Methode und Ergebnis [Developing Dementia friendly Organizations through participatory research. Participation as means and ends.]. In F. L. Uribe, S. Kuliga, M. Roes, & S. Teupen (Eds.), *Partizipative Forschung mit Menschen mit Demenz. Chancen und*

Herausforderungen für die qualitative Forschung. Beiträge aus dem MethodenForum Witten 2022 [Participatory research with people with dementia. Chances and challenges in qualitative research. Contributions from the MethodenForum witten 2022]. Beltz Juventa.

Thalén, L., Malinowsky, C., Margot-Cattin, I., Gaber, S. N., Seetharaman, K., Chaudhury, H., Cutchin, M., Wallcook, S., Anders, K., Brorsson, A., & Nygård, L. (2022). Out-of-home participation among people living with dementia: A study in four countries. *Dementia, 21*(5), 1636–1652. https://doi.org/10.1177/14713012221084173

von Unger, H. (2012). Partizipative Gesundheitsforschung: wer partizipiert woran? Participatory Health Research: Who Participates in What? Investigación participativa en salud: ¿Quién participa en qué? http://nbn-resolving.de/urn:nbn:de:0114-fqs120176

Ward, R., Clark, A., Campbell, S., Graham, B., Kullberg, A., Manji, K., Rummery, K., & Keady, J. (2018). The lived neighborhood: Understanding how people with dementia engage with their local environment. *International Psychogeriatrics, 30*(6), 867–880. https://doi.org/10.1017/S1041610217000631

Woodbridge, R., Sullivan, M. P., Harding, E., Crutch, S., Gilhooly, K. J., Gilhooly, M. L. M., McIntyre, A., & Wilson, L. (2018). Use of the physical environment to support everyday activities for people with dementia: A systematic review. *Dementia, 17*(5), 533–572. https://doi.org/10.1177/1471301216648670

Zepke, G., & Finsterwald, M. (2022). *Evaluierung des Projektes "Eine Bibliothek für Alle- die demenzfreundliche Bibliothek Wiener Neustadt"* [Evaluation of the project 'A library for All - the dementia-friendly library Wiener Neustadt.] Unpublished report.

8

Rural and urban transportation and technology use

What needs to be considered?

Sarah Wallcook, Camilla Malinowsky and Anna Brorsson

Introduction

Globally the number of older people aged 65 years has increased and is estimated to be 1.5 billion in 2050 (United Nations, 2019) while the number of people with dementia in the same year is estimated to be 131.5 million (Prince et al., 2015). All people, including people living with dementia, should have equal rights to full participation and inclusion in society (Shakespeare et al., 2019). To uphold these rights, different initiatives need to be taken and developed, for example, age-friendly communities, which seek to promote equality, participation and dignity in an ageing society (Buckner et al., 2019; Plouffe & Kalache, 2010). Another such initiative is active ageing, which is about optimising opportunities for participation, health and security to enhance quality of life. Age-friendly communities involve designing services, structures and environments that are accessible and inclusive to older people living with varying disabilities, preferences and needs (World Health Organization, 2007). A related concept is dementia-friendly communities, which focus on adapting services and structures to be inclusive and accessible for active ageing (Cutler & Kane, 2006) and promote social inclusion and community participation for people with dementia (Marsh et al., 2018). This concept seeks to enable people with dementia to enact a sense of agency and to remain active and independent (Innes et al., 2011; Wiersma, 2008). Achieving such a vision means that community-based services and businesses should consider the needs and preferences of people with dementia as citizens to create and offer cultural, leisure and recreational activities that promote community engagement (Buckner et al., 2019; Marsh et al., 2018).

Involvement of people with dementia

This chapter is based on research that used walking interviews in an action research methodology in Stockholm, Sweden, and home-based interviews in a rural part of northern England. The European Working Group of People

DOI: 10.4324/9781003416241-12

with Dementia, and a local Focus on Dementia Network group consulted on the data collection and analysis phases and discussed the findings of the UK-based studies.

Travelling, technology and community engagement

Doing activities outside home is contingent on reaching, and thereby, going to a particular place in the community. Different modes of transport can be used, e.g. walking that is being a pedestrian (Brorsson et al., 2011, 2013, 2016), using public transport or transportation services (Brorsson et al., 2011) or driving a car (Hansen et al., 2020; Rapoport et al., 2020). People with dementia tend to do activities near home (Brorsson et al., 2011; Duggan et al., 2008) with the neighbourhood being a place that is more strongly retained over time while engagement with other types of places reduce (Gaber et al., 2023; Thalén et al., 2022). Furthermore, when going to places further away from home, people with dementia often make the journey together with other people (Brorsson et al., 2011, 2013). However, what constitutes as 'far' can vary according to where you live, as, for example, people living in rural communities often need to make longer journeys in order to reach friends and family members and undertake basic activities such as grocery shopping and doctor's appointments (Wallcook et al., 2022). Furthermore, the unique geography, population density and distances involved in travelling in rural places create poor conditions for effective public transportation, so that driving is often the only viable option (Rapoport et al., 2020). Consequently, people with dementia living rurally drive for longer than people living in urban areas (Spinney et al., 2020). Furthermore, if that travelling becomes impossible, community engagement drastically reduces and a person may be forced to find a new home closer to the people, places and activities that are central to everyday life (Spinney et al., 2020; Wallcook et al., 2024).

With respect to making journeys, people with dementia experience many different problems related to doing activities outside home, for example, finding the way, locating signs and timetables and interpreting and using this information (Brorsson et al., 2011, 2013, 2016, 2020). Moreover, the increasing ubiquity of technology in everyday life is changing how people make journeys and engage with places outside home (van Holstein et al., 2022). For example, buying travel and parking tickets less often occurs in a face-to-face customer services exchange and is more likely to occur via an everyday technology (i.e. ticket machine, travel or payment card machine and reader). These technologies can vary considerably in design and increasingly require people to use their own mobile or download a smartphone application. Possibly due to differences in design features and siting between and within different countries, these types of technologies encountered outside home are typically more challenging to use and their difficulty varies (Wallcook et al., 2020). As users of these technologies, people with dementia have been shown to overlap with matched groups of people with no known cognitive impairment in terms of the amount of technologies used and ability to them (Wallcook et al., 2020; Wallcook, Nygård, Kottorp, & Malinowsky, 2021). However, people with dementia often face increasing difficulties over time where a reduction in technology use also relates to a reduction in the places people go to outside home (Hedman et al., 2018; Wallcook, Nygård, Kottorp, Gaber, et al., 2021).

Using vignettes from our research, we highlight the interplay between travelling and technology in rural and urban contexts and discuss emerging issues and innovations.

Vignettes

Rural Cumbria

Michael lives alone and drives 10 kilometres from his small village with no shops to the closest supermarket on the outskirts of town almost every day. One reason for making the trip so often is that Michael abandons his shopping before it is complete as he is concerned about the consequences of overstaying in the carpark. The landowner has subcontracted the carpark management to a third-party company that uses automatic numberplate recognition technology to support enforcing a maximum stay of two hours. The design features of this technology are minimal in terms of the feedback they provide to the driver parking the car. There is no direct interaction with the technology, no ticket, or display that the driver can check to verify their time of arrival or how long they are allowed to stay. Instead, the driver must remember to check and monitor their own time of departure independently. The rules for using the carpark and consequences of overstaying are displayed on signboards with dense text. Furthermore, the driver receives no immediate notification of a fine, instead this arrives by post to their registered address after the fact. Within this technologised parking system, there is no option for Michael to make a payment to extend his parking and ensure sufficient time to complete the tasks at hand. Previous experience and ongoing concerns that he would fail to abide by the rules mean that Michael adapts his activities and routines and frequents the supermarket more often to finish the unfinished shopping. In other settings however, Michael opts for technological over face-to-face interactions as they provide visual feedback and focus between him and the technology without distraction from other people. Technologies that let him see information, such as instructions and payment amounts on screen, mean that Michael experiences greater control, lack of distraction and security in paying at the pump and using automated check-outs than he does using face-to-face customer services. Michael is therefore willing to drive further distances to reach places, such as petrol stations, that offer his preferred match of technologies.

Urban Stockholm

Sue lives alone in a city apartment. When participating in out-of-home activities, concerns could start in the home. She has to remember what to bring, e.g. a wallet, shopping list or travel card and this can result in mental fatigue even before going outside home which affects how she experiences the accessibility and usability of public space. When doing activities outside home she usually travels by public transportation such as the subway, commuter train or bus. To make such a journey she needs a ticket and uses a travel card with the option to load money because she does not travel often and does not need a monthly travel card. Sue has several concerns about this travel card. One concern is when she needs to load the card with money. This can be done at a ticket machine at the stations and that means that she has to interact with the machine. This situation is experienced as challenging since she finds it difficult to follow the instruction on the display and it also requires that she have some pre-knowledge about how to use the machine. It is not only the interaction with the ticket machine that makes it difficult, but also what is going on in the surrounding environment. She avoids situations where there is a long queue to the machine as this situation makes her very stressed and it becomes even harder to use the machine. That is, she can interact with the machine when she can do it at her own pace and when there is no queue behind her. Another concern is that she feels unsure whether the ticket is valid during the journey, which occurs mainly when she changes mode of public transportation and when the time for the journey is longer. This can result in checking the ticket several times at the ticket counter so that she has a valid ticket in order not to get caught in ticket control. She has considered where she put her travel card and that she can access it easily. She has a specific place in her handbag where she puts it. Now she is waiting for her 'free travel pass' [färdtjänstkort] which will facilitate her travels as she does not need to worry that she has money on the travel card, and will always have a valid ticket. With this card, she will travel for free with public transportation and she does not have to worry about economic issues related to transportation.

Implications for the development of cognitively inclusive communities

Beware digitalisation as the source of new problems

These vignettes point towards a shared drive for efficiency and effectiveness through technology in both rural UK and urban Sweden, and how this is creating fewer opportunities for people with dementia to approach a person for a service or to ask for help. The vignettes illustrate how this fuels concern both in using transport and parking services, and in meeting the demands of the technologies that replace a face-to-face service. In both contexts, the upshot is that digitalisation has increased the demand on the travellers' preparedness and pre-knowledge of what is needed to undertake the journey, including how to use the technologies that will be encountered. For people who know that they may not be able to respond spontaneously to the situation at hand, this means planning before leaving home, undertaking practice runs, and checking for changes that impact the plan (Brorsson et al. 2011).

Changes can occur suddenly which travellers need to respond to, for example, a new technology can be installed, or an older more familiar technology replaced. Unexpected diversions on familiar routes and public transport lines, changes to road and station layouts, relocation of bus stops, can also challenge travellers with dementia to a greater extent than travellers whose cognition provides a problem-solving and orientation advantage. In combination, our vignettes highlight how these challenges can lead to repeated attempts, missed appointments, late arrival, stress, and disorientation, which disadvantage and negatively impact people with dementia.

Design and provide cognitively inclusive travel technologies

Aspects of cognitive inclusivity extend to how travel technologies and systems are designed to provide, or not provide, feedback about time. In the situations described for the Sweden and UK vignettes, the onus is currently being placed on the traveller to remember how long the public transport ticket is valid, or how long the car has been parked. In particular, the useability of Intelligent Travel Systems monitoring length of parking stay through, e.g. Automatic Number Plate Recognition is seriously hampered by not providing feedback to the user. Furthermore, many car parking facilities are removing on-site ticket machines in favour of smartphone applications, which users are required to download and use. These applications have been designed with little attention to inclusive use and various recommendations have been made to improve useability. For example, providing notification support with expiry times and options to extend the parking, and providing a support mode tailored to disabled drivers' needs (Paiva et al., 2023). An aspect of the Stockholm public transport system that supports cognitive accessibility is that the exit gates are automated by passing through rather than needing to use a ticket (Wallcook et al., 2020). In the UK, the ticket or contactless payment card often needs to be produced at entry and exit, which can entail remembering to seek out the exit touchpoint where failure to do so incurs a maximum daily charge. However, Stockholm public transport tickets are limited to 75 minutes of journey time which may lead travellers to be concerned about incurring a penalty if their journey is delayed due to dementia-related issues such as taking a wrong connection or needing extra time. Consequently, the cognitive inclusivity of travel technologies with respect to time orientation need to be improved to mitigate the increased likelihood that a person with dementia will fall foul of a penalty or fine.

Living up to future promises

Driving cessation is a reality at some point on the trajectory of living with dementia, and autonomous vehicles are increasingly described as saviours for people living with dementia to continue driving (Haghzare et al., 2023). However, the rural vignette illustrates that people with dementia can be driving their vehicle without mishap and instead the problems that impact travelling can first arise when using a parking technology. Parking the car should not involve excessive technological demands that unduly and adversely impact someone's possibility to drive thereby imposing barriers in everyday life. Neither should difficulties using an unfamiliar technology be conflated with hazardous driving of a familiar vehicle (Byszewski et al., 2013). Moreover, for autonomous vehicles to achieve their hoped-for impact, cognitively inclusive parking solutions are an essential prerequisite.

Disability parking permits could provide an inclusive solution and in the UK these permits have been made available to people with dementia on the grounds of severe psychological distress, being at risk of harm or experiencing difficulty or inability to walk (Hare, 2019). However, these permits do not apply in all carparks (i.e. on private land), and the focus remains on proximity of parking as the goal. This means the badge is not targeted to support the prominent cognitive issues raised by the rural vignette, such as attention, orientation in time and the memory and executive functioning demanded by on-site parking technologies.

In concert, the urban vignette highlights how using the public transport system can be facilitated by providing a free travel pass with unlimited validity. In statistical studies, concessionary public transport provision has been seen to associate with going to a greater number of places, reduced loneliness and increased contact with friends and children (Gaber et al., 2020; Reinhard et al., 2018). A travel pass could be combined with a range of other public transport innovations, such as colour-coded signage to support wayfinding, staff awareness training, Try Before You Ride initiatives, and a commitment to continue providing face-to-face services (van Holstein et al., 2022). Collectively, these initiatives could drastically reduce the cognitive demands otherwise posed by the public travel system and related technologies, opening the door to sustained community engagement for people with dementia.

Conclusion

This chapter spotlights the interplay between transportation options and technology use as often-neglected aspects of initiatives targeted towards cognitively inclusive community engagement. Involving people with dementia to take a holistic view of problematic travel and technology situations that arise outside home helps to identify the limits of innovations. Particularly helping to identify in advance where an innovation may create new issues rather than solve existing problems. As human progress continues at pace, there is an urgent and ongoing need to address the cognitive inclusivity of all aspects of communities, including transportation solutions and technology design.

In-depth box

- The interplay between transportation and technology use is a critical, but often neglected part of dementia-inclusive communities.
- Our knowledge on this topic is generated with people with dementia through participatory action research and consultation on the planning, analysis and reporting of the studies.
- New initiatives and innovations need to take a broad view and involve people with dementia in transport technology design to eliminate the risk of unintentionally creating new problems.
- Cognitive inclusivity should lie at the heart of community development and the drive for sustainable human progress.

References

Brorsson, A., Öhman, A., Cutchin, M., & Nygård, L. (2013). Managing critical incidents in grocery shopping by community-living people with Alzheimer's disease. *Scandinavian Journal of Occupational Therapy, 20*(4), 292–301. https://doi.org/10.3109/11038128.2012.752031

Brorsson, A., Öhman, A., Lundberg, S., Cutchin, M. P., & Nygård, L. (2020). How accessible are grocery shops for people with dementia? A qualitative study using photo documentation and focus group interviews. *Dementia, 19*(6), 1872–1888. https://doi.org/10.1177/1471301218808591

Brorsson, A., Öhman, A., Lundberg, S., & Nygård, L. (2011). Accessibility in public space as perceived by people with Alzheimer's disease. *Dementia, 10*(4), 587–602. https://doi.org/10.1177/1471301211415314

Brorsson, A., Öhman, A., Lundberg, S., & Nygård, L. (2016). Being a pedestrian with dementia: A qualitative study using photo documentation and focus group interviews. *Dementia, 15*(5), 1124–1140. https://doi.org/10.1177/1471301214555406

Buckner, S., Darlington, N., Woodward, M., Buswell, M., Mathie, E., Arthur, A., Lafortune, L., Killett, A., Mayrhofer, A., Thurman, J., & Goodman, C. (2019). Dementia friendly communities in England: A scoping study. *International Journal of Geriatric Psychiatry, 34*(8), 1235–1243. https://doi.org/10.1002/gps.5123

Byszewski, A., Aminzadeh, F., Robinson, K., Molnar, F., Dalziel, W., Man Son Hing, M., Hunt, L., & Marshall, S. (2013). When it is time to hang up the keys: The driving and dementia toolkit – for persons with dementia (PWD) and caregivers – a practical resource. *BMC Geriatrics, 13*(1), 117. https://doi.org/10.1186/1471-2318-13-117

Cutler, L. J., & Kane, R. A. (2006). As Great as All Outdoors. *Journal of Housing for the Elderly, 19*(3–4), 29–48. https://doi.org/10.1300/J081v19n03_03

Duggan, S., Blackman, T., Martyr, A., & Van Schaik, P. (2008). The impact of early dementia on outdoor life: A 'shrinking world'? *Dementia, 7*(2), 191–204. https://doi.org/10.1177/1471301208091158

Gaber, S. N., Nygård, L., Kottorp, A., Charlesworth, G., Wallcook, S., & Malinowsky, C. (2020). Perceived risks, concession travel pass access and everyday technology use for out-of-home participation: Cross-sectional interviews among older people in the UK. *BMC Geriatrics*, *20*(1), 192. https://doi.org/10.1186/s12877-020-01565-0

Gaber, S. N., Nygård, L., Malinowsky, C., Brorsson, A., Kottorp, A., & Hedman, A. (2023). Enacting citizenship through participation in a technological society: A longitudinal three-year study among people with dementia in Sweden. *Ageing and Society*, *43*(2), 276–297. https://doi.org/10.1017/S0144686X21000544

Haghzare, S., Stasiulis, E., Delfi, G., Mohamud, H., Rapoport, M. J., Naglie, G., Mihailidis, A., & Campos, J. L. (2023). Automated vehicles for people with dementia: A "tremendous potential" that "has ways to go"—Reports of a qualitative study. *The Gerontologist*, *63*(1), 140–154. https://doi.org/10.1093/geront/gnac115

Hansen, S., Newbold, K. B., Scott, D. M., Vrkljan, B., & Grenier, A. (2020). To drive or not to drive: Driving cessation amongst older adults in rural and small towns in Canada. *Journal of Transport Geography*, *86*, 102773. https://doi.org/10.1016/j.jtrangeo.2020.102773

Hare, P. (2019). How can we really make the Blue Badge work for people with dementia? Retrieved from http://www.innovationsindementia.org.uk/2019/06/how-can-we-really-make-the-blue-badge-work-for-people-with-dementia/

Hedman, A., Kottorp, A., Almkvist, O., & Nygård, L. (2018). Challenge levels of everyday technologies as perceived over five years by older adults with mild cognitive impairment. *International Psychogeriatrics*, *30*(10), 1447–1454. https://doi.org/10.1017/S1041610218000285

Innes, A., Kelly, F., & Dincarslan, O. (2011). Care home design for people with dementia: What do people with dementia and their family carers value? *Aging & Mental Health*, *15*(5), 548–556. https://doi.org/10.1080/13607863.2011.556601

Marsh, P., Courtney-Pratt, H., & Campbell, M. (2018). The landscape of dementia inclusivity. *Health & Place*, *52*, 174–179. https://doi.org/10.1016/j.healthplace.2018.05.013

Paiva, S., Amaral, A., Pereira, T., & Barreto, L. (2023). Conceptual architecture for an inclusive and real-time solution for parking assistance. In E. G. Nathanail, N. Gavanas, & G. Adamos (Eds.), *Smart energy for smart transport* (pp. 1083–1091). Springer Nature Switzerland. https://doi.org/10.1007/978-3-031-23721-8_88

Plouffe, L., & Kalache, A. (2010). Towards global age-friendly cities: Determining urban features that promote active aging. *Journal of Urban Health: Bulletin of the New York Academy of Medicine*, *87*(5), 733–739. https://doi.org/10.1007/s11524-010-9466-0

Prince, M., Wimo, A., Guerchet, M., Ali, G.-C., Wu, Y.-T., Prina, M., & Alzheimer Disease International. (2015). *World Alzheimer Report 2015 The global impact of dementia: An analysis of prevalence, incidence, cost and trends*. London: Alzheimer Disease International. Retrieved from https://www.alzint.org/u/WorldAlzheimerReport2015.pdf

Rapoport, M., Hyde, A., & Naglie, G. (2020). Transportation issues in dementia. In A. Innes, D. Morgan, & J. Farmer (Eds.), *Remote and rural dementia care: Policy, research and practice* (pp. 213–240). Bristol: Policy Press.

Reinhard, E., Courtin, E., Van Lenthe, F. J., & Avendano, M. (2018). Public transport policy, social engagement and mental health in older age: A quasi-experimental evaluation of free bus passes in England. *Journal of Epidemiology and Community Health*, 72(5), 361–368. https://doi.org/10.1136/jech-2017-210038

Shakespeare, T., Zeilig, H., & Mittler, P. (2019). Rights in mind: Thinking differently about dementia and disability. *Dementia, 18*(3), 1075–1088. doi:10.1177/1471301217701506

Spinney, J. E. L., Newbold, K. B., Scott, D. M., Vrkljan, B., & Grenier, A. (2020). The impact of driving status on out-of-home and social activity engagement among older Canadians. *Journal of Transport Geography, 85*, 102698. https://doi.org/10.1016/j.jtrangeo.2020.102698

Thalén, L., Malinowsky, C., Margot-Cattin, I., Gaber, S. N., Seetharaman, K., Chaudhury, H., Cutchin, M., Wallcook, S., Anders, K., Brorsson, A., & Nygård, L. (2022). Out-of-home participation among people living with dementia: A study in four countries. *Dementia, 21*(5), 1636–1652. https://doi.org/10.1177/14713012221084173

United Nations (2019). *World Population Ageing 2019.* New York: United Nations Department of Economic and Social Affairs, Population Division Highlights. Retrieved from https://www.un.org/en/development/desa/population/publications/pdf/ageing/WorldPopulationAgeing2019-Report.pdf

van Holstein, E., Wiesel, I., & Legacy, C. (2022). Mobility justice and accessible public transport networks for people with intellectual disability. *Applied Mobilities, 7*(2), 146–162. https://doi.org/10.1080/23800127.2020.1827557

Wallcook, S., Malinowsky, C., Charlesworth, G., Ryd, C., & Nygård, L. (2024). Everyday technology's interplay in the lives of people with dementia: A multiple case study in the rural North of England. *Journal of Rural Studies, 106*, 103203. https://doi.org/10.1016/j.jrurstud.2024.103203

Wallcook, S., Malinowsky, C., Nygård, L., Charlesworth, G., Lee, J., Walsh, R., Gaber, S., & Kottorp, A. (2020). The perceived challenge of everyday technologies in Sweden, the United States and England: Exploring differential item functioning in the everyday technology use questionnaire. *Scandinavian Journal of Occupational Therapy, 27*(8), 554–566. https://doi.org/10.1080/11038128.2020.1723685

Wallcook, S., Nygård, L., Kottorp, A., Charlesworth, G., & Malinowsky, C. W. (2022). Conditions of technology use and its interplay in the everyday lives of older adults with and without dementia. In M. Orrell, D. Oliveira, O. McDermott, F. R. J. Verhey, F. C. M. Dassen, & R.-M. Dröes, *Improving the lives of people with dementia through technology* (1st ed., pp. 73–85). Routledge. https://doi.org/10.4324/9781003289005-9

Wallcook, S., Nygård, L., Kottorp, A., Gaber, S., Charlesworth, G., & Malinowsky, C. (2021). Kaleidoscopic associations between life outside home and the technological environment that shape occupational injustice as revealed through cross-sectional statistical modelling. *Journal of Occupational Science, 28*(1), 42–58. https://doi.org/10.1080/14427591.2020.1818610

Wallcook, S., Nygård, L., Kottorp, A., & Malinowsky, C. (2021). The use of everyday information communication technologies in the lives of older adults living with and without dementia in Sweden. *Assistive Technology: The Official Journal of RESNA, 33*(6), 333–340. https://doi.org/10.1080/10400435.2019.1644685

Wiersma, E. C. (2008). The experiences of place: Veterans with dementia making meaning of their environments. *Health & Place, 14*(4), 779–794. https://doi.org/10.1016/j.healthplace.2008.01.001

World Health Organization. (2007). *Global age-friendly cities: A guide.* France: World Health Organization. Retrieved from https://www.who.int/ageing/publications/Global_age_friendly_cities_Guide_English.pdf

9

Toilets

A key feature for inclusive design. Newbuild and refurbishment

Gill Mathews, Mary Marshall and Heather Wilkinson

Introduction

This chapter addresses the issue of toilet design for older people with dementia, an issue that requires careful attention, but which is often neglected. Here, we consider reasons for the common lack of oversight and its potential consequences, drawing on co-produced research on public toilets to illustrate key points. Design enhancements are proposed for both new buildings and refurbishment. We also highlight the importance of adopting a human rights approach when planning for inclusive provision.

Lack of attention in toilet design

Toilet design for people with dementia is often neglected. This leads to problems with accessibility and siting. Different reasons for such inattention include attitudinal influences; equipment vagaries and modifications; regulatory factors; maintenance and refurbishment; and a lack of training for those involved in toilet creation.

Toilets are private spaces for carrying out ablutions and eliminating body waste but human beings have varied, complex and personal viewpoints when it comes to attending to these aspects of behaviour and the matter often evades open discussion. Haslam (2012), for example, in his book *Psychology in the Bathroom* asserts that, 'despite its importance, excretion is something that people rarely want to think about, instead we try to put the greatest possible distance between ourselves and our waste' (p. 2). Bringing the topic into the public domain is, however, important to normalise what is an essential and natural process of being human. Adopting a positive and pragmatic approach will help to change the attitudinal mind-set and facilitate a more honest and inclusive debate around toilet needs.

The equipment used in toilets is subject to frequent change. This is partly a fashion issue, partly a technology issue, partly a materials issue. Collectively, these factors greatly influence what is available and at what cost. Other regulatory factors, such as infection control, are prioritised by designers but,

DOI: 10.4324/9781003416241-13

without forward thinking about the potential range of consumers and their different needs, can have an adversarial impact on usability due to impractical features. For example, taps conceived to prevent the spread of infectious disease are often too complex and difficult to decipher for a person living with a cognitive impairment (British Standards Institution, 2022).

Washroom and toilet components require regular maintenance and replacement due to the moist atmosphere and repeated use. Refurbishment, therefore, offers the opportunity to increase toilet accessibility. Unfortunately, without due consideration, this can lead to new unhelpful features being installed. Toilets are usually accorded low priority in the building design process with important details frequently omitted from the main design brief. Ensuing mistakes can be hard to remedy, resulting in inferior and non-inclusive provisions. Designers need adequate training to support a clear focus on the preferences of divergent users and to give attention to the ways in which people with different needs might interact with technology. Attention to safety issues and optimal positioning of the various toilet constituents are essential aspects. Although most countries will specify design requirements for a standard disabled toilet (e.g., Standards Australia, 2021), additional critical features to enable ease of use for people with dementia and many older people, are habitually overlooked. Siting is another important factor. People with dementia need the toilet to be easy to find and easy to use (Marshall, 2022), yet, in many buildings, toilets evade discovery due to concealed siting and inadequate signage.

Consequences

Every one of us needs to be able to find and use a toilet if we are to function as normal citizens. It is a vital human right. Without suitable toilet access, autonomy, and the potential to go outdoors, are curbed. Things that many of us take for granted become impossible. This applies to all areas in public use: shopping streets and shops, places of worship, public galleries, restaurants and cafes, hotels; transport, etc. Ensuring toilets are accessible in hospitals and care homes is necessary as inhabitants are usually those who experience the most acute vulnerability as a result of illness, frailty and dementia (Healy & Shanahan, 2022). A report from the Geller Institute of Ageing and Memory (National Institute for Health Care and Research, 2022) found very high use of incontinence pads for people with dementia in acute hospital wards. For many, this was linked to a failure to find and access the toilet. Simple measures can, however, make a huge difference to increase independence, confidence and dignity. A good example of this is when one nursing home for people with dementia halved the use of incontinence pads merely by making the toilet doors more visible to residents. The doors were painted in a contrasting colour to the adjacent walls and given a visible sign with clear lettering so that they were easily discovered and understood.

The inability to understand and cater for peoples' basic needs is a serious issue that can carry fateful consequences including feelings of shame and distressed behaviour. Ignorance often adds insult to injury, e.g. the use of the term 'wanderer', sometimes given by care staff to those who walk around seeking the toilet, shows a lack of training and recognition of the underlying cause (Marshall & Allan, 2006). Hospitals and care homes have a duty of care to ensure that staff are adequately educated and that they are providing appropriate toilet provisions when they are caring for people with vulnerabilities. It is all too easy to blame the dementia diagnosis and overlook the key issue of poor comprehension and deficient toilet design and access.

Generally, the need for uncomplicated toilet access becomes more of an issue as we age. Anxiety about not being able to find or use a toilet prevents many older people from venturing outside, restricting freedoms to engage in activities that others may take for granted. People with dementia mostly fall within the older age bracket and are, therefore, more likely to experience conditions associated with ageing, e.g. urgency linked to pelvic floor muscle weakness, prostate problems and frequency resulting from commonly prescribed medications such as diuretics.

Above, we have outlined some of the main reasons to impress why enabling toilet design and siting are key factors in maintaining self-respect and well-being for people with dementia. The next section explores some of these issues using a case study of a recent research project entitled, "A Public Inconvenience" (Mathews et al., 2022).

A case study – a public inconvenience

This case study presents the findings from a project that explored the everyday challenges faced by people with dementia and other disabilities needing to use a toilet whilst travelling. Working with people with lived experience as co-researchers, the specific objectives were to: (1) gather relevant data on transport-related toilet provision in Scotland; and (2) highlight key issues and make recommendations for inclusive toilet provision to transport industry policymakers, planners and design specialists. By presenting the case study within this chapter we seek to highlight the importance of accessible toilet provision as an integral aspect of people's daily lives. Ong et al. (this volume) include a perspective on this project from a person with lived experience.

The starting point for the work was a recognition that for people living with dementia and other physical and cognitive impairments, the quality and accessibility of public toilet provision when travelling in the United Kingdom (UK) is a major issue. As previously mentioned, talking about going to the toilet can be a private and sensitive topic. Inhibitions about airing toilet needs prevent widespread discussion and, consequently, taking the necessary actions to promote social inclusion that good toilet access can underpin (Marshall, 2022). The inadequacy of toilet provision and poor design means that many people are left feeling frustrated, sad, angry and excluded due to an inability to enjoy activities that most of us take for granted (Slater & Jones, 2018; Tales et al., 2017). There are more than 230,000 people in the UK who require personal assistance to use the toilet, yet few of the standard accessible toilets meet these needs (Grant, 2013). Despite an acknowledgement by Scotland's Accessible Travel Framework (Transport Scotland, 2016) that accessible toilets are a fundamental aspect of Human Rights (HR), toilet provision for people whilst travelling continues to be a significant problem. A failure to meet British Standards for building is a common feature. There are two UK-wide standards, issued by the British Standards Institute (BSI), that affect toilet design in Scotland: BS6465 parts 1–4 and BS8300 (British Standards Institution, 2018). Despite no legal obligation to meet these standards, compliance signals organisational diligence.

What we did: Researchers from the Edinburgh Centre for Research on the Experience of Dementia (ECRED) and community partners – DEEP (Dementia Engagement and Empowerment Project), the Dementia Centre, HammondCare, PAMIS (Promoting a more inclusive society), Upstream (explores the challenges of mobility and travelling with dementia) – worked alongside people with disabilities including dementia and other physical and cognitive impairments. Carers of people with profound and multiple learning disabilities were also involved. We used a qualitative, co-production design, to ensure an inclusive approach (Pernia et al., 2021). The photographic method was used, based on the work and ethos of PhotoVoice Hamilton (2007) who promote the participatory and ethical use of photography for positive social change. Our research aim was to identify the specific needs and key shared priorities that require to be addressed to enable people with dementia and other impairments to use toilet facilities while travelling. The research took place over eighteen months and was structured across three phases, each punctuated by a 'Gathering'. The 'Gatherings' acted as critical events that brought together the participant co-researchers (PCO) and project partners at key junctures, to facilitate:

Gathering 1: Information sharing, recruitment and PCO training (Month 3)
Gathering 2: Collective data analysis, preparing the knowledge exchange and impact plan (Month 10)
Gathering 3: Staging an event to disseminate findings (Month 15)

Gatherings were held in Aberdeen and Edinburgh to support recruitment across Scotland. Eleven PCOs took part. Data were collected from city and rural locations around Scotland including airports, bus and railway stations and motorway service stations. Some 'destinations' such as museums and cinemas were also included.

Data took the form of photographs, verbal recordings and/or short videos accompanied by written descriptions. The latter were encapsulated in photo-diaries which provided a standardised framework for data collection (Table 9.1 below). The PCOs captured elements of toilet accessibility and design that were problematic and/or helpful to them and described their felt experience.

Over 1,000 photographs were created by the PCOs. These covered 86 locations across nine Scottish regions and included bus and rail stations and ferry and airport terminals.

The findings were captured in four main themes:

Theme 1: Difficulties accessing the toilet. It can be hard to find, get in and get out of a public toilet

The PCOs' found that toilets are often difficult to find, tucked away, out of sight. The problem is not helped by poor signage and dark lighting (refer BSI 8300, Sections 12 and 14) (British Standards Institution, 2018). Signs are often too high up, too small or not clear. Figure 9.1 (below) illustrates an example of clear signage.

Another challenge when looking for a toilet was the lack of available facilities. It was not uncommon to discover a toilet that was locked or out of order with no indication about where else to go. Change machines also produced concerns. Most of the machines encountered were positioned too high for a wheelchair user to reach. In some toilets, it was necessary to have the right coinage to enter a toilet. It can be a very complex task for someone with a cognitive impairment to decipher the instructions on these machines which are often in very small writing.

Table 9.1 Photo diary template

Name:	Location:	Date:
WHAT DO YOU NOTICE?	**HOW DOES IT MAKE YOU FEEL?** (for example: uncomfortable? Safe? Anxious?)	
Finding the toilet – are they easy to find? What do you notice about the signage? What do you **see**? (how is the lighting? Are surfaces or reflections unhelpful?) What do you **hear**? (are there loud noises? Confusing noises?) What do you **smell**? (does the environment smell pleasant? Are there artificial scents?) How **easy** is it to use? (operating taps, opening doors, locking and unlocking...) How **helpful** are people? Anything else that you notice...		

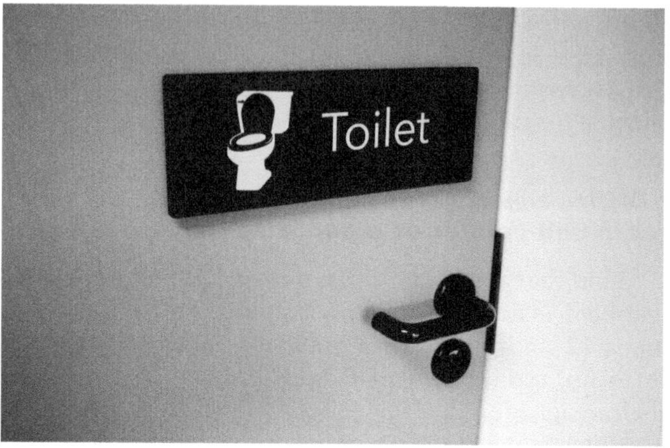

Figure 9.1 Example of a good, clear toilet sign.

Theme 2: Ease of use public toilets can present a major challenge to use

Disabled people often need a good amount of space in which to move around but the PCOs reported that many public toilet spaces, including 'accessible' toilets, were often too small to facilitate ease of movement, especially for wheelchair users. This may be because many of the toilets included in this study met standards that were current when they were built – but which are no longer compliant. There was rarely sufficient space for the use of large, non-contact bins for continence pads. The problem is frequently exacerbated through clutter (some toilets are used as storage spaces), poor design and layout of equipment. Sinks that are too small often splash water; equipment such as hand-driers, air fresheners and heaters often look similar, making it hard for anyone to work out which is which. Further, the positioning of these can make them problematic to use, e.g. hand-driers that are hard to reach. Buttons, without any accompanying label, compound this matter and it was not uncommon for the toilet user to be uncertain as to whether a door was locked or unlocked, again prompting anxiety.

Theme 3: Emotional distress. Using public toilets can be distressing

Many of the sights, sounds, smells and physical encounters with toilets were upsetting to the PCOs, especially those with sensory impairments. Some of the PCOs experience visual challenges, and some with dementia have the additional challenge of perceptual problems (Houston & Christie, 2018). This means that they misinterpret what they are seeing – for example, moving from darker to lighter flooring can be perceived as a step, increasing the risk of a fall.

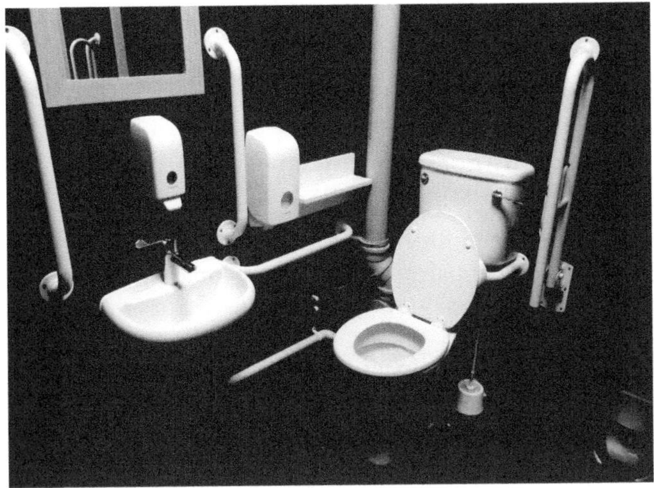

Figure 9.2 Clear contrast of all essential features in a toilet.

For the ageing eye and those with other visual challenges, a clear contrast in tone (Figure 9.2) is crucial if they are to see important features of a toilet – a white basin on a white wall and pale floor is, for example, invisible. Other essential features such as the toilet roll holder also need to contrast with the wall if they are to be seen.

A wide range of physical challenges were reported by the PCOs working on this project. They also described how they felt when faced with difficulties. Many of the toilets were hard to find, unwelcoming, dirty and poorly maintained, sometimes with no staff in attendance to offer support. This resulted in feelings of distress and a sense of exclusion. The relationship between unpleasant physical experiences and emotional anguish was clearly evidenced, highlighting the acutely negative impacts of sensory overload.

Theme 4: Universal and unique needs: needs identified mainly overlapped but there were some key differences

People with a variety of physical and cognitive impairments, and carers of people with profound and complex needs came together to co-create the study, describing and documenting their experience of toilets when travelling. The process of being involved raised individual PCO awareness about the wider spectrum of issues beyond their own needs. They told us that it was rewarding to be involved with others and to learn about different needs, some of which were highly visible whilst others were not openly observed. The advantage of carrying out surveys within a group context was that everyone had a slightly different outlook and experience, creating rich and varied data.

Based on the research findings, the next section provides a brief summary of the essential requirements, identified by the PCOs that enable people with dementia to find and use a toilet.

Getting it right – understanding the impairments for which design has to compensate

Clearly no toilet will be tailor-made for an individual except perhaps within their own home but the impairments of most people with dementia which can be assisted by improved design that gives focused attention to the impact of:

- Impaired memory (helped by visibility and signage)
- Impaired problem-solving (easy access/ simple to use)
- Impaired learning (simple to use)
- Sensory difficulties (care with lighting, contrast, sound, smell, etc.)

The majority of people with dementia are in the later stages of life, therefore the normal impairments of this phase require to be addressed. These include, for example, a need for adequate lighting as well as strong contrast of key features specifically a light reflectance value of 40L (Bowes et al., 2014; Mc-Nair & Pollock, 2017). Additionally, older people tend to stoop more and have more pronounced muscle weakness. This can be helped by raising the height of the toilet and also avoiding push-button flush systems.

Getting it right – finding the toilet

Finding the toilet requires good signage using identifiable graphics and simple words to lead the intended user directly to the toilet door.

Signage is a major issue for people with dementia. Essentially, the symbols and the words used on toilet signs need to be clearly understood. Modern toilet signage is generally based on internationally agreed conventions using male and female stick figures (International Organisation for Standardisation (ISO), 2023). Some people with dementia will have difficulty understanding these symbols partly because they do not indicate that there is a toilet. Similarly, a wheelchair graphic does not tell people that there is a toilet. For many the word 'toilet' will be sufficient but for people who have lost the ability to read or whose first language is not English, a clearly understood graphic depicting a toilet is critically important. The words on toilet signs also require to be well-defined to maximise legibility, particularly for people with impaired vision. Barker and Fraser (2000) recommend the use of capital letters at the start of each word followed by lower case and a large font without serifs. Contrast is an important factor to ensure that the words and graphics are distinct against the background. The sign itself requires to be differentiated from its background and mounted at an accessible height. The same principles apply to the toilet door which needs to be clearly distinguished from wall in which it is sited, both inside and outside. The sign needs to be visible on the door, not adjacent or above and an exit sign on the inside of the toilet door can be very helpful, especially if there are other doors such as cupboard doors. In the case of new builds in a hospital or care home, the toilet door should be evident from where people commonly sit, e.g. in the lounge and dining room. In the bedroom, it should be observable from the bed. (Namazi & Johnson, 1991). Modern methods of ventilation mean that there is a lot less of a problem with unpleasant smells emitting from toilets in hospitals and care homes.

Signage and identifying the door can easily be achieved as part of refurbishment but the current lack of suitable signage pinpoints these as key areas for attention.

Getting it right – the room itself

Careful design and positioning of toilet equipment within the washroom promotes accessibility.

On entering the toilet, prominent positioning of the toilet pan ensures immediate recognition. Again, contrast is central to ensure that the different features, e.g. wash hand basin and grab rails, are clearly demarcated against the walls and floor.

With regards to equipment, simplicity and familiarity are critical enablers. Strange taps, soap dispensers, toilet paper holders and flush controls can be confusing and may even cause distress. Toilet fixtures and fittings are constantly changing and what appears typical to younger generations may be hard to decipher for an older person with dementia. The problem can be addressed by adopting tried and tested designs that are readily recognisable and have utility across the age range. Account also needs to be given to cultural norms – what is regarded as customary in one country may differ across nations, e.g. mixer taps have been common in Australia for many years so are likely to be less alien to a person with dementia as they would be in the UK.

In some rarer forms of dementia, people can lose their comprehension of what a mirror is and are unable to recognise their own reflection. Instead, there is a perception that someone else, a stranger, is in the room with them. This scenario is, understandably, extremely distressing. Ideally, in such instances, it should be possible to pull down a blind or obscure the mirror when using the toilet. Perceptual problems may also result in people misapprehending patterns on the floor, wall tiles or other wall coverings, e.g. jazzy patterns can look as if they are moving, and speckled floor coverings can appear dirty (Houston & Christie, 2018).

Moving forward, attention to these features can be included in new-build facilities, and particularly in those places where there is a higher percentage of usage by people with dementia such as acute hospitals and care homes.

The approach needed

A human rights approach to address citizen needs is increasingly being adopted. People who live with impairments are entitled in law to enabling design that facilitates their access to experiences in the same way (or as similar as possible) as other citizens. In most industrialised nations, for example, the wheelchair lobby has ensured awareness of their particular needs in toilet design and, in the UK, we have a British Standard for disability BS8300 (British Standards Institution, 2018). The requisites of people with other types of impairments are, however, often neglected.

Positively, dementia is now accepted as a disability in formal documents and legislation. This means that people with dementia have citizen rights which are enshrined under both the UK Equality Act 2010 and the 2006 United Nations Convention on the Rights of Persons with Disabilities (CRPD). The Equality Act covers every kind of disability and does include enabling design. In 2019 the UK All Party Group Parliamentary on Dementia published their report: *Hidden no more. Dementia and disability* which covered every aspect of the lives of people with dementia. The report did not, however, focus on design. Encouragingly, the publication of the new Publicly Available Standard on designing for neurodiversity (British Standards Institution, 2022) does refer to the needs of people with dementia. With an ageing society and increasing numbers of people living longer with this condition notice needs to be given to the overall quality of life experience and to what actions are required to ensure that equal access for all moves beyond the slogan to become a tangible reality.

Concluding remarks

Within the UK, there is a growing understanding that people with dementia live with a disability and that they are therefore entitled to dignity, independence and participation. The availability of well-designed toilets is a key enabler within this respect but, unless appropriate action is taken, these citizen rights continue to be unfulfilled. This brief chapter has raised some of the main issues relevant to inclusive toilet design as described by people with lived experience who researched the topic. Their findings and perspectives reinforced our existing concerns. Here, we offer a starting point for guidance on some essential features of facilitative design. Our hope is that this important area of work will be given greater credence in the future so that the design of toilets will achieve the urgent attention it deserves.

In-depth box

- Designing to ensure that people with dementia can find and use a toilet is essential if they are to remain as independent as possible and to participate in society as fellow citizens.

- This chapter emphasis this as a Human Rights issue and describes the consequences of failing to attend to the needs of people with dementia. An account of original, co-produced research into the provision of toilets whilst travelling is included.
- The chapter briefly provides information about necessary design requirements. There is an emphasis on hospitals and care homes, although the chapter is wider in its application.

References

Barker, P., & Fraser, J. (2000). *Sign design guide: a guide to inclusive signage.* Sign Design Society and RNIB.

Bowes, A., McCabe, L., Dawson, A., & Greasley-Adams, C. (2014). *Design of living spaces for people with dementia and sight loss.* Pocklington Trust.

British Standards Institution. (2018). BS8300–2:2018 Design of accessible and inclusive built environment. Buildings. Code of practice. In. United Kingdom: BSI.

British Standards Institution. (2022). PAS 6463 Design for the mind – neurodiversity and the built environment – Guide. In. United Kingdom: BSI.

Grant, A. (2013). *Changing places: the practical guide.* Changing Places Consortium.

Photovoice Hamilton. (2007). Manual and resource kit. *Hamilton, Ontario: Hamilton Community Foundation.* Retrieved April 4, 2024 from: https://www.naccho.org/uploads/downloadable-resources/Programs/Public-Health-Infrastructure/Photovoice-Manual.pdf

Haslam, N. (2012). *Psychology in the bathroom.* Springer Verlag London.

Healy, M., & Shanahan, M. (2022). Continence. In C. Cunningham, M. Healy, & S. Macfarlane (Eds.), *BPSD textbook: addressing behaviours and psychological symptoms of dementia.* HammondCare.

Houston, A., & Christie, J. (2018). *Talking sense. Living with sensory changes and dementia.*

International Organisation for Standardisation (ISO). (2023). *ISO 7001:2023(en) Graphical symbols — Registered public information symbols.* ISO. Retrieved June 12, 23 from, https://www.iso.org/obp/ui/#iso:std:iso:7001:ed-4:v1:en

Marshall, M. (2022). *Toilet talk. Accessible design for people with dementia* (2nd ed.). HammondCare.

Marshall, M., & Allan, K. (2006). We walk, they wander. In G. Stokes (Ed.), *Dementia: walking not wandering. Fresh approaches to understanding and practice.* Hawker Publications.

Mathews, G., Marshall, M., & Wilkinson, H. (2022). A public inconvenience: better toilets for inclusive travel. *Disability & Society, 37*(7), 1146–1172.

McNair, D., & Pollock, R. with Cunningham, C. (2017). *Enlighten. Lighting for older people and people with dementia* Sydney, Dementia Centre HammondCare.

Namazi, K. H., & Johnson B. D. (1991). Physical environmental cues to reduce the problems of incontinence in Alzheimer's disease units. *American Journal of Alzheimer's Disease and Other Dementias, 6*(6), 22–28.

National Institute for Health Care and Research. (2022). *Continence, dementia, and care that preserves dignity.* NIHR. Retrieved June 12, 2023, from https://evidence.nihr.ac.uk/themedreview/continence-dementia-and-care-that-preserves-dignity/

Pernia, R., Haya, S., & Salmón, I. (2021). Inclusive research, learning disabilities, and inquiry and reflection as training tools: a study on experiences from Spain. *Disability & Society, 36*(6), 978–998.

Slater, J., & Jones, C. (2018). *Around the Toilet: a research project report about what makes a safe and accessible toilet space.* Sheffield Hallam University.

Standards Australia. (2021). AS 1428.1:2021 Design for access and mobility, Part 1: General requirements for access - New building work. In. Australia: Standards Australia.

Tales, A., Burholt, V., Nash, P., Bichard, J. A., & Clayton-Turner, A. (2017). Dementia-friendly public toilets. *Lancet, 390*(10094), 552–553. https://doi.org/10.1016/s0140-6736(17)31813-5

Transport Scotland. (2016). *Going further: Scotland's accessible travel framework.* Edinburgh: Scottish Government. https://www.transport.gov.scot/media/20113/j448711.pdf

Selected innovative research projects I

Introduction

This chapter describes two innovative research projects by early-career researchers that add novel perspectives, innovative research methods, and personal reflections on their lessons-learnt to the current discourse of dementia and design.

These contributions reflect on designing the built and/or social environment based on the perspectives of people living with dementia – *and together with them*. Two further innovative research projects relating to the care home environment are included as Chapter 17 of this volume.

1 The first contribution, authored by Janissa Altona, Henrik Wiegelmann, Emily Mena, Julia Misonow, Christoph Teves, Benjamin Schüz, and Karin Wolf-Ostermann describes preliminary results of a literature analysis, wayfinding study, and participatory stakeholder workshops, to derive meaningful input for urban planners.
2 The second contribution, by Saskia Kuliga, Martina Roes, and dementia advocate Jim Mann describes a participatory co-research project, in which people living with dementia evaluated spatial orientation and wayfinding in their living environments; not as study participants, but as co-researchers and collaborators.

DOI: 10.4324/9781003416241-14

Project 1

Dementia-enabling neighbourhoods – participatory development of dementia-enabling neighbourhoods in Bremen

Janissa Altona, Henrik Wiegelmann, Emily Mena, Julia Misonow, Christoph Teves, Benjamin Schüz and Karin Wolf-Ostermann

Background

Physical barriers and resources in the neighbourhood-built environment (NBE) can play a crucial role for community-dwelling people living with dementia (PlwD) when it comes to their physical, psychological, social, and cognitive health (Chen et al., 2022). Basically, studies indicate that having an NBE that is designed to be as barrier-free as possible contributes to PlwD's ability to remain physically and socially active, which in turn has a positive impact on mental and cognitive health (Gan et al., 2020). Similarly, the World Alzheimer's Report (2020) emphasizes the role of the built environment and makes a *"strong statement that design for dementia is 30 years behind the physical disabilities movement – and that this must change."*

In this contribution, we present the main elements of the ongoing innovative pilot project ("DEN-HB – Dementia-Enabling Neighbourhoods: Participatory Development of Dementia-Friendly Neighbourhoods in Bremen") as well as preliminary results. The project is currently ongoing and still being implemented in the city of Bremen (Germany), where it aims to contribute to improved dementia-friendly NBEs.

Experimental approach

This study is designed as a mixed methods study and is made up of the three following main components:

1 Umbrella Review: A systematic literature review was conducted as an umbrella review (Altona et al., 2022). The aim of the review was to search and summarize known NBE factors as important aspects for the design of dementia-friendly neighbourhoods.
2 360-Degree Wayfinding-Study: A cross-sectional validation study in the urban area of Bremen, (Germany) using Apple Maps Street View (2020/22) with a 360-degree viewing angle is aimed.

DOI: 10.4324/9781003416241-14

3 Participatory Stakeholder Workshops, focus groups, and individual interviews: to discuss the results and implications of the study with family carers of PlwD, and PlwD, among others, and to propose recommendations for action.

Preliminary results

The following key criteria – based on elements of the ecological model of cognitive health by Cerin (2019) – were identified via the Umbrella Review as influential for the dementia-friendliness of NBE structures (Table 10.1).

Results of the review show that the aspect of wayfinding infrastructure plays a key role in qualitative studies and that there are still gaps in research. Therefore, the 360-degree wayfinding-study was planned in which a standardized, quantitative questionnaire was developed based on the following thematic criteria:

- General streetscape
- Complexity of the public traffic area
- Footpaths, bicycle paths, motorways
- Public transport stops
- Practical, aesthetic, and natural design elements
- Buildings
- Signage

Five urban districts with a high proportion of older residents (>65 years) in the city of Bremen were chosen and at least two randomly selected geo coordinates were drawn for each street within these districts to collect data on wayfinding structures (Figure 10.1) with the help of the developed questionnaire.

Table 10.1 Key criteria

Aspect of the neighbourhood-built environment	Examples
Green and blue infrastructure	Parks, forests, public gardens, lakes, rivers
Mixed land use	Mix of building types with various uses (e.g. residential buildings, cafés, stores)
Density	Population density, building density
Street network connectivity	Connections, crossings, dead ends
Pedestrian and bicycle infrastructure	Bike paths, sidewalks
Transportation infrastructure	Roads for buses, tracks for trains, ports, airports
Physical disorder	Neglected buildings and land, vandalism
Wayfinding infrastructure	Signage, markings, acoustic signals

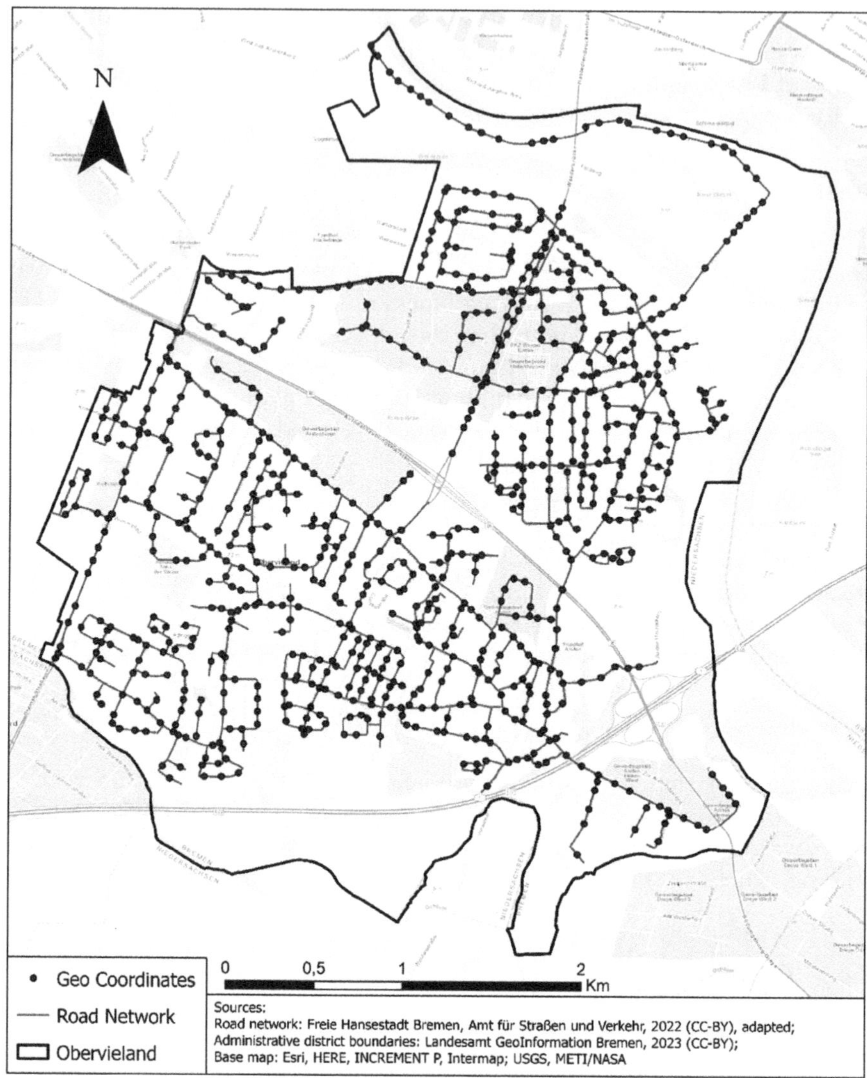

Figure 10.1 GIS-Map of randomly selected geo coordinates of the district Obervieland, Bremen.

Furthermore, context data is provided, such as street noise. The data evaluation is conducted within and between the city districts in comparison. Apple Maps Street View and its 360-degree perspective were utilized for this survey.

Conclusions

In order to provide meaningful input for urban planning, research projects such as the present one need to systematically interact with key stakeholders in urban health. Following best practice examples for the dissemination and validation of dementia-friendly city concepts (Pozo Ménendez et al., 2022), the steps will include discussing and validating the results in participatory workshops with experts from practice, science, and self-advocacy initiatives and reaching a consensus on recommendations for action to promote dementia-friendliness in the city of Bremen.

The implementation of the 360-degree viewing method via digital maps employs an innovative survey method that could drive future research on the relationship between orientation-promoting aspects of the built environment and dementia, also independently of hard-to-reach target groups, such as PlwD. The project results provide a useful triangulation of important NBE factors for PlwD and their presence or absence in the urban context allows a good basis for participatory urban planning of dementia-friendly cities.

In-depth box

- One part of the DEN-HB research project uses Apple Maps (Street view) by randomly selecting roundabout 3,000 geo-coordinates from the city of Bremen (Germany).
- We plan participatory research through workshops, focus groups, and individual interviews with PlwD and/or their relatives.
- The innovative approach of the 360-Dregree Wayfinding-Study also fulfils sustainable aspects, as resources can be saved in data collection. In addition, the form of data collection has the potential to be extended to national and international levels without the need for researchers to be present in the field.

Funding statement

The project is funded by the Tönjes-Vagt Foundation in Bremen.

References

Altona J, Wiegelmann H, Mena E, Schüz B, Wolf-Ostermann K (2022). Associations between neighbourhood-built environment and cognitive or social health among people with dementia. Results of an Umbrella Review in the Project Dementia-Enabling Neighbourhoods: Participatory Development of Dementia-Friendly Neighbourhoods in Bremen (DEN-HB), 32. Alzheimer Europe Conference 2022, Bucharest, Romania, 19 October 2022

Cerin E (2019). Building the evidence for an ecological model of cognitive health. Health Place. 2019, 60:1–3. Doi: 10.1016/j.healthplace.2019.102206

Chen X, Lee C, Huang H (2022). Neighborhood built environment associated with cognition and dementia risk among older adults: A systematic literature review. Soc Sci Med. 2022 Jan;292:114560. Doi:10.1016/j.socscimed.2021.114560

Gan DRY, Chaudhury H, Mann J, Wister AV (2021). Dementia-friendly neighbourhood and the built environment: A scoping review. Gerontologist. 2021 Feb 10:gnab019. Doi:10.1093/geront/gnab019

Freie Hansestadt Bremen, Amt für Straßen und Verkehr (2022) (CC-BY), adapted; Administrative district boundaries: Landesamt GeoInformation Bremen, 2023 (CC-BY); Base map: Esri, HERE, INCREMENT P, Intermap; USGS, METI/NASA

Pozo Menéndez E, Higueras García E (2022). Best practices from eight European dementia- Friendly study cases of innovation. Int J Environ Res Public Health. 19:14233. Doi:10.3390/ijerph192114233

Project 2

Inclusive co-research with people living with dementia about wayfinding in their living environment and neighbourhood

Saskia Kuliga, Martina Roes and Jim Mann

Dementia-sensitive built environment – where and how we started

The ambition driving the INCLUDE research project was to start a participatory action research group with a co-creative method toolkit based on qualitative research-, design thinking- and wayfinding research methods. As interdisciplinary researchers, we sought to evaluate, together with co-researchers living with dementia, how they orient themselves in- and experience their living environments. By living environment, we mean the residential place, but also the connecting neighbourhood and city one lives in: the holistic environment, in which all daily human-environment and lifeworld-related interactions take place.

INCLUDE set the perspective of people living with dementia as co-researchers central. Hence, they were both study participants as well as co-researchers who were invited to engage in decisions about the project's research focus. The research topic was spatial orientation and wayfinding in urban environments, as this is one of the relevant aspects of a dementia-sensitive built environment from the perspective of people living with dementia (Rohra & Mann, et al., 2021). Also, we invited the co-researchers to bring in their own topics related to how they perceive, experience and interact with the built environment.

In our methodological toolbox, at the start of the project, we had planned situated wayfinding evaluations, photovoice methods, cultural probe methods, and co-creative design thinking methods, with facilitated discussions about the experiences of the co-researchers about their living environment (cf. Brannelly & Bartlett, 2020; Gaver et al., 2004; O'Connor et al., 2020; White & Devitt, 2021). Co-researchers could choose which environment they wished to evaluate, e.g. their home or neighbourhood. Overall, this approach resulted in qualitative (audio) data, including photos, and memos from personal observations. We focused on the research question, what would strengthen navigational confidence during wayfinding from the perspective of the co-researchers living with dementia.

DOI: 10.4324/9781003416241-14

For the remainder of this short contribution, we share personal reflections and informal observations. As this is an ongoing research project, at the time of writing, we have not yet formally analysed the qualitative data. Hence, all of the following insights are preliminary, and we share personal observations:

Preliminary insights about the methods and form of the participatory research project

An important lesson we learnt was that it was challenging for us, as researchers, to get in touch with people living with dementia who were motivated to engage in this type of study and who lived at different locations. Also, the form we initially chose, the participatory action research group with people living with dementia, was a new approach for both the individuals living with dementia and the associated agencies and facilitators.

The final co-researcher sample consisted of four people living with dementia who participated several times, and two groups of two, respectively, three individuals who joined as a group of people who already knew each other. During some of the research meetings, familiar people, such as a family member or a social worker, acted as facilitators. All co-researchers and two project collaborators lived with early stages of dementia (one dropped out due to scheduling difficulties).

The four individual co-researchers participated in between two and six meetings. The two groups of two, respectively, three co-researchers engaged in one situated wayfinding evaluation and a subsequent seated interview about the experience and methods, whereas the individual co-researchers engaged in all methods we had prepared. Overall, a participatory action research group could not be set-up as originally planned, leaving the primary source of input one-on-one discussions with the co-researchers. This choice was the co-researchers' preference to form the participatory research meetings.

Sharing informal lessons learned about the method toolkit that we had envisioned at the start of the project, we first must note that the method we used most often were seated- or walking interviews. These were situated in the familiar living environment or a familiar urban environment. Hence, we did not use the full range of methods we had prepared within the methodological toolbox. For example, despite having prepared the cultural probe methods (such as co-creative design tasks, e.g., taking pictures with a single-use camera, using maps, or diaries), the co-researchers did not choose these themselves, unless we explicitly asked them to use these. However, *when* they chose to take photos during the situated wayfinding evaluations, this seemed to be an enjoyable task for them. Taking pictures by themselves appeared to support the co-researchers in reflecting about the situated wayfinding and environmental evaluations.

We noted that the co-researchers opened-up to share personal experiences about their perspectives the most, when the research was given form as informal conversation, when the researcher also shared personal data about herself, or when there was an easy atmosphere with, e.g., something to eat or drink on the table, before talking about the research topics.

Preliminary insights about the research focus: what have we learnt?

A few directions where the project could take us are already visible and we can present these as preliminary personal observations:

First, we learned that spatial orientation and wayfinding were not the sole focus of people living with dementia when the co-researchers talked about it conceptually. Nevertheless, during the situated wayfinding evaluations, it was quite clear to the researcher accompanying the walks, that spatial orientation was indeed important. Co-researchers were able and navigationally confident to identify shortest routes when they were familiar with the environment. Yet, it was sometimes hard to predict directions to global landmarks (such as a church), when these were not visible; and local landmarks were unique to the particular wayfinder (such as an object or place that was meaningful for them individually). Overall, co-researchers identified routes towards the destinations they wanted to reach, talked about it with self-reflection, and enjoyed the situated wayfinding evaluations.

Second, the co-researchers reflected on how they would make decisions, and, as is also supported by other studies, co-researchers chose and preferred familiar routes and –areas. Yet, each of the nine individual co-researchers participating in INCLUDE also had an individual perspective on what was important for them in their interactions with the built environment. For instance, they had different ways of dealing with situations in which they had to (re-)orient themselves. This is not surprising, given that people who do not live with dementia also have individual wayfinding strategies and preferences, and that assessing these in research requires quite nuanced perspectives about the individual wayfinder (Carlson et al., 2010; Kuliga et al., 2019). This makes generalization for research purposes difficult, but also offers novel avenues of thinking about the users of the built environment in a nuanced way.

Third, we did experience brief moments during the data collection, when a co-researcher momentarily was not able to orient themselves. These moments lasted seconds to a few minutes only. They were linked to short-lived strong emotional reactions and meant we paused the study at these times. The researcher who accompanied the situated wayfinding evaluations could not have predicted these moments. It is sometimes difficult to disentangle the dynamic effects that might have caused the disorientation, since we relied on qualitative data (audio recordings). Yet, in retrospect, we might interpret that these disorienting moments occurred when the co-researcher decided either already had walked for an extended time and perhaps was cognitively fatigued, or when we had spontaneously to enter an unfamiliar part of an environment, with full navigational confidence that this would not pose any challenge.

Our next steps include analysing all collected data and diving deeper into the interpretation of the project's results. This includes considering recommendations for environmental planning stakeholders and – designers and further understanding of the different methods for the involvement of people living with dementia in research focused on the built environment (also cf. Fahsold et al., 2023). Our long-term vision is to bridge the perspectives of the different stakeholders involved in the theoretical and practice-oriented discourse on dementia and environmental design research. This might also foster sustainable design solutions (Kuliga et al., 2021), with people living with dementia at the heart and centre thereof.

In depth box

- The INCLUDE project had a participatory action research focus. We invited people living with dementia as co-researchers and collaborators on eye-level, to evaluate, together, how they experienced the built environment they lived in, and how they oriented and engaged in wayfinding.
- Preliminary insights of this ongoing research project indicate that each co-researcher living with dementia had a unique, individual focus of what was important to them when evaluating the built environment. Wayfinding and spatial orientation were important aspects when evaluating the built environment and embedded within their *holistic* experience of the living environment.
- By including insights on the perspectives of people living with dementia in research, these perspectives will be visible in the research literature. Environmental planners/designers might reach sustainable design solutions, when taking these perspectives as the starting point and core of their design decisions.

Acknowledgments

We thank all co-researchers who had the courage to raise their voice and participated in this research endeavour, as well as all facilitators, practical supporters and collaborators.

Ethics

The project received ethical approval by Deutsche Gesellschaft für Pflegewissenschaft, registered as Nr. 22–008, in Germany.

Funding Statement

The research project INCLUDE is funded by "Deutsche Demenzhilfe – DZNE Stiftung für Forschung und Innovation" within the "Innovative Minds" program.

References

Brannelly, T., & Bartlett, R. (2020). Using walking interviews to enhance research relations with people with dementia: Methodological insights from an empirical study conducted in England. *Ethics and Social Welfare, 14*(4), 432–442. https://doi.org/10.1080/17496535.2020.1839115

Carlson, L. A., Hölscher, C., Shipley, T. F., & Dalton, R. C. (2010). Getting lost in buildings. *Current Directions in Psychological Science, 19*(5), 284–289. https://doi.org/10.1177/0963721410383243

Fahsold, A., Roes, M., Holle, B., & Kuliga, S. (2023). Methods for the involvement of people living with dementia in research focused on the built environment: A protocol for a scoping review. *BMJ Open, 13*(8), e075350. https://doi.org/10.1136/bmjopen-2023-075350

Gaver, W.W., Boucher, A., Pennington, S., & Walker, B. (2004). Cultural probes and the value of uncertainty. *Interactions, 11*(5), 53–56. https://doi.org/10.1145/1015530.1015555

Kuliga, S., Berwig, M., & Roes, M. (2021). Wayfinding in people with Alzheimer's disease: Perspective taking and architectural cognition—A vision paper on future dementia care research opportunities. *Sustainability, 13*(3), 1084. https://doi.org/10.3390/su13031084

Kuliga, S. F., Nelligan, B., Dalton, R. C., Marchette, S., Shelton, A. L., Carlson, L., & Hölscher, C. (2019). Exploring individual differences and building complexity in wayfinding: The case of the Seattle central library. *Environment and Behavior, 51*(5), 622–665. https://doi.org/10.1177/0013916519836149

O'Connor, D., Phinney, A., Mann, J., Chaudhury, H., Seetharaman, K., Landy, A., & Paulina, M. (2020). Living with dementia: Flipping stigma on its ear. *Innovation in Aging, 4*, 41–42. https://doi.org/10.1093/geroni/igaa057.135

Rohra, H., Mann, J., Rommerskirch-Manietta, M., Roes, M., & Kuliga, S. (2021). Wayfinding and urban design from the perspective of people living with Dementia–A call for participatory research. *Journal of Urban Design and Mental Health, 7*(4), 1–18. https://www.urbandesignmentalhealth.com/journal-7-wayfinding.html

White, P. J., & Devitt, F. (2021). Creating personas from design ethnography and grounded theory. *Journal of Usability Studies, 16*(3). https://doi.org/10.1007/978-3-031-05412-9_2

General hospital design

Dementia-friendly hospitals

Current state and future directions

Suzanne Timmons and Emma O'Shea

Introduction

Acute hospital admission is typically intended as a short-term stay, focused on assessing and treating/managing urgent medical needs, which cannot be addressed in other healthcare settings at that time. Given the acute care focus, 'dementia' is not usually the primary reason for admission (Bracken-Scally et al., 2020), and the presence of dementia is often not given due consideration in terms of care planning and delivery. This is problematic, because in recent years we have determined that 20–40% of hospital admissions aged 65+ have dementia (Briggs et al., 2017; Morandi et al., 2019; Timmons et al., 2015). It is also known that a significant proportion of people with undiagnosed dementia remain undiagnosed during hospital admissions (Brady et al., 2016), indicating poor awareness and recognition of the condition. Given changing demography and trends towards population aging, the prevalence of dementia amongst hospital inpatients will continue to rise and health systems must adapt accordingly.

Acute dementia care is costly (Carter et al., 2023; Reynish et al., 2021), and health policies in many Western countries (e.g., UK, Ireland, Netherlands) are focused on reducing the rates of avoidable hospital admissions for this cohort. Unfortunately, the policy-practice gap persists, as funds are not being sufficiently redirected into the development of robust community-based health and social care services (Prince et al., 2016; Toot et al., 2013). Hospital-based dementia care is also impacted upon by organisational structures, including a workforce employed to attend to acute healthcare needs, in a timely and cost-efficient manner. The behaviour of healthcare staff in acute settings tends to align with the acute care goals, rather than considering the individual differences of dementia patients (Chenoweth et al., 2021; Houghton et al., 2016), because they are incentivised and reinforced to do so by organisational structures and culture.

This chapter will consider the role of the social and physical aspects of the hospital environment in dementia care, drawing on data relating to outcomes of hospital admission; experiences of care recipients and their family

DOI: 10.4324/9781003416241-16

carers; data reflecting current care practices and policies; perspectives of care providers, including barriers and facilitators of person-centred care; evidence for environmental interventions and quality improvement initiatives; and directions for future research.

Outcomes of hospital admission

Failure to address the psychosocial, occupational, and environmental needs of people living with dementia may contribute to the known range of adverse outcomes in this cohort, including lengthier hospital stays (Carter et al., 2023; Reynish et al., 2021), increased risk of mortality (Lehmann et al., 2018; Rao et al., 2016; Reynish et al., 2017, 2021), institutionalisation (Lehmann et al., 2018), hospital readmission (Reynish et al., 2021), and functional decline (Pedone et al., 2005; Reynish et al., 2021).

Delirium superimposed on dementia (DSD) is another significant factor to consider, since people with dementia are up to six times more likely to be admitted to hospital with delirium (Ahmed et al., 2014). The evidence demonstrating the high prevalence of DSD amongst hospital inpatients (approx. 49–57%) (Han et al., 2022; Timmons et al., 2015) has led some to suggest that it is not useful to consider dementia and/or delirium in isolation (Reynish et al., 2017), and instead we should be considering cognitive impairments in a more global manner, i.e., 'cognitive spectrum disorders'.

Patients with DSD have significantly worse outcomes. For example, a recent systematic review and meta-analysis (Han et al., 2022) found DSD was significantly associated with greater length of hospital stay, cognitive and functional decline, and a higher risk of institutionalisation and mortality, compared to patients with dementia, without delirium. Importantly, our 'INAD-2' audit (Bracken-Scally et al., 2020) showed that while over half of hospitals in Ireland with an emergency department stated that they screen 'some or all' patients for delirium, only 19% of patients with dementia had evidence of delirium screening in their healthcare records (HCRs).

Another factor of note includes the high rate of new prescriptions of antipsychotic medication for patients with dementia during hospital admissions (Timmons et al., 2023). The risks associated with antipsychotic use in dementia are well-established (Nørgaard et al., 2022). Despite this, antipsychotic use for managing non-cognitive symptoms of dementia (NCSD) persists. Timmons et al. (2023) found, via HCR review of inpatients with dementia, that new/increased antipsychotic medication was prescribed for NCSD in approximately 12–18% of the total patient cohort (N = 893).

Experiences of hospital care

The evidence relating to how hospital admissions are experienced by people with dementia and their families, unsurprisingly points to many areas for improvement, especially in relation to the physical and psychosocial environment.

A qualitative review of seven included studies by Reilly and Houghton (2019) focused on hospital experiences of people with dementia specifically, via the theoretical lens of Brooker's 'VIPS' framework (Values, Individualised approach, Perspective of person with dementia, Social environment) (Brooker & Latham, 2015). Key findings included the experience of care being 'rushed' and primarily task-focused, with poor and 'paternalistic' staff communication, leaving patients feeling ignored and excluded. Hospital environments were considered unsuitable (e.g., noisy, crowded, inappropriate lighting, poor signage), contributing to distress which exacerbated NCSD, sometimes leading to physical and chemical restraint use (e.g., for 'wandering'; 'aggression'). The authors note that both observational studies and patients' qualitative accounts indicated that noisy climates and a frantic pace within the environment worsened disorientation, and reduced patients' sense of control and independence. Having shared toilet facilities, a lack of privacy, and inability to control lighting/noise levels were especially agitating and disempowering. Hallways were sometimes cluttered with equipment (e.g., machines, linen trolleys) which raised safety issues and rendered wayfinding even more challenging.

Conversely, there were times when patients were under-stimulated; boredom was noted as a 'commonality' across studies, linked to a lack of meaningful engagement. This, according to the review authors, highlights the need for dementia training/education, and staff supervision and support, to facilitate reflection on dementia care practices and environmental design in their own setting. Finally, the authors emphasise the importance of incorporating the perspectives of people with dementia in the design and remodelling of hospital spaces, in line with previous authors' recommendations (Digby & Bloomer, 2014; Topo et al., 2012). More recent studies, not included in Reilly and Houghton's (2019) review, further reinforce the above findings, and highlight continued deficits in relation to the provision of person-centred dementia care in hospitals (Chenoweth et al., 2021; Scerri et al., 2020).

Hospitalised people with dementia are typically (though not always) supported closely by relatives, who can provide valuable information for staff about the patient, which becomes increasingly important as the condition advances. Unsurprisingly, hospital admissions can also be intense and distressing experiences for family members (Burgstaller et al., 2018; Keuning-Plantinga et al., 2021). Burgstaller et al. (2018) conducted a systematic review and meta-ethnography (n = 12 studies) exploring the experiences and needs of family members during hospital admissions. Although there were some positive experiences reported, the experiences were predominantly negative. Key concerns of family members related to the poor suitability of the busy hospital environment, which some indicated exacerbated NCSD. Another key concern was the lack of dignity-supporting care interactions, which indicated to family members that staff are not always adequately trained to provide appropriate dementia care. In line with the evidence from the perspectives of people with dementia, family carers also experienced the care approach as 'task-oriented' and were often disappointed and angered by the lack of attention from staff. Carers reported that communication from staff about care was poor throughout the admission, leaving them feeling ignored, undervalued, and stressed.

Characterising 'dementia-friendly' hospitals

Over the last decade, in particular, the idea of 'dementia-friendly' hospitals (DFHs) has gained traction, as one part of the wider 'dementia-friendly' movement.

Manietta et al. (2022) conducted an integrative literature review (N = 34 papers), characterising current descriptions of DFHs. The authors identified six characteristics of DFHs, i.e., (i) care continuity, (ii) person-centeredness, (iii) consideration of phenomena within dementia, (iv) the physical hospital environment, (v) valuing relatives, and (vi) knowledge and expertise within the hospital. The authors point out that the term 'dementia-friendly' is more often used in quality improvement projects, rather than in research publications based on empirical studies. Furthermore, they state that perspectives of people with dementia are rarely included. While these findings are intuitive and useful at individual and interpersonal levels, they don't consider the entire hospital ecosystem as a setting driven by culture, policies, and systems.

Parke et al. (2017) point to the potential utility of the 'social-ecological model' for characterising the 'fit' between people with dementia and hospital environments; a model which Parke and Chappell (2010) had previously used in a critical ethnography focused on hospitalised older adults more generally. This model assumes that people cannot be understood in isolation from their environmental context. The environmental context in this instance is physical, social, and organisational; all three must be considered to determine what contributes to eventual outcomes. Parke and Chappell (2010) outline the following interrelated factors as central to the person-hospital fit, i.e., (i) social climate, (ii) physical design, (iii) care systems and processes, and (iv) policies and procedures. They argue that if these four factors are optimised for the provision of person-centred dementia care, then this can be considered a 'dementia-friendly' hospital.

While the evidence from the perspectives of patients and family carers focused significantly on the poor suitability of the social climate, physical design, and the task-focused nature of the care systems/processes, there was (naturally) little focus on policies and procedures, or on systemic factors that contribute to care cultures. To gain a more holistic understanding, we must also consider: (1) dementia care policies and practices at various levels of the hospital environment, and (2) other stakeholders' (i.e., healthcare workers') perspectives on dementia care provision, to provide context for staff behaviour and patient/family experiences. This will be achieved in the following two sections by (1) drawing on our recent national audit data, and (2) examining barriers to optimal care provision from the provider perspective.

Evaluating dementia care practices and policies

In 2019, the second Irish National Audit of Dementia Care in Acute Hospitals (Bracken-Scally et al., 2020) was conducted to generate current data on care policies and practices and to monitor progress since round one. The audit tools, originally developed for the 'England and Wales Audit of Dementia Care in Hospital Settings' (Royal College of Psychiatrists, 2011) were designed to measure key criteria relating to care delivery, which are known to impact on people with dementia admitted to hospital. With permission from the original audit group, we replicated this audit in the Republic of Ireland, making minor modifications to the tools to ensure they were fit-for-purpose in the Irish setting. The second round of audit data (INAD-2) was based on 33 hospitals nationally and had three distinct components, i.e., the 'organisational' audit (hospital-level: policy and processes); a HCR review (patient-level: actual practice, N = 934) and the 'environmental' audit (ward-level). Some key findings at hospital-level include that just 6% of hospitals had a dementia care pathway in place and under one-quarter had a dementia recognition system in place. More positively, 85% of hospitals stated they provide dementia awareness training, which was an improvement on INAD-1.

In relation to the physical environment, most hospitals reported having implemented some dementia-friendly environmental changes. Still, INAD-2 found that only a small proportion of wards (N = 72) had adequate environmental cues to aid orientation. Just one-quarter of wards had colour schemes in use, and this was compounded by insufficient and/or inappropriate signage. For example, there was signage on 'some or all' toilet doors in 76% of wards audited. Few wards (17%) had space (outside of the ward corridor) for people with dementia to walk in, and just under half of wards provided handrails along the corridors to facilitate this. Where handrails were observed, they were sometimes obstructed by hospital equipment. The flooring in most hospital wards was appropriate for the visual needs of a person with dementia, in terms of plain/subtle pattern and subtle polish. Just over half of wards (53%) had a room/area available for patients and families to use for social purposes, or as a break from the busy ward environment.

It is also worth detailing INAD-2 findings relating to psychosocial care elements, and the overall person-centredness of the care approach. For example, the use of 'patient passports', or other documents which collect personal information pertinent to providing a tailored approach to care, was evidenced in just 2% of HCRs reviewed (17/934). Despite depression being common in this cohort, just 11% of patients had any assessment of mood during their admission. There was poor access to social and therapeutic activities, with just 42% of hospitals (14/33) having these in place. Furthermore, communication with family carers was poor across several indices, including poor recording of collateral history relating to the nature of the dementia progression (31%) and relating to behaviour changes consistent with NCSD (23%). Communication was poor in other respects also, echoing the findings outlined above from carers' perspectives. For instance, just 61% (193/319) of HCRs indicated that an assessment of the family carer's needs had taken place in advance of discharge (where relevant); while only 28% of HCRs (185/664) indicated any advanced notice of discharge. The patterns in these findings validate the experiences of people with dementia and family carers. However, they don't give us insight into why the provision of optimal dementia care in hospital environments can be so challenging.

Barriers: the provider perspective

There have been several literature reviews focused on the provider perspective on hospital dementia care, and the associated barriers, including inadequate dementia awareness training; cultures that (i) prioritise physical needs and (ii) inhibit information-sharing, either with patients/families, or between hospital staff; and inappropriate physical environments which are busy and chaotic, and which don't support orientation, wayfinding, social interaction, or meaningful activity (Gwernan-Jones et al., 2020; Houghton et al., 2016; Turner et al., 2017).

Duah-Owusu White and Kelly (2023) recently published a narrative review exploring staff views on hospital dementia care across 33 qualitative papers, using a 'systems approach'. The findings provide context for the experiences of patients and family carers, as well as the above audit data. Staff sometimes experience people with dementia as aggressive or hostile, and in the absence of a patient's ability to communicate verbally, staff are often unable to interpret the meaning of behaviours. Some reported that this makes it difficult to meet patients' needs and to forge positive relationships. Patient safety is a major priority for staff. This is mandated at hospital-level, and staff indicate that where potential patient risks are identified, a risk reduction approach would override any competing patient preferences.

Staff must also contend with the potential financial and legal implications of decisions relating to patient care, as well as meeting requests from other hospital and community-based colleagues. Staff acknowledge the value of input from family members, and that this knowledge and expertise is not always sufficiently mined. Some indicated that communicating with families can create more work that is not directly relevant to the patient's acute care needs (e.g., assuaging family fears/anxieties). Furthermore, complex family dynamics can complicate care decisions, rather than assist them, particularly when staff believe that a family member's perspective is not grounded in the patient's best interest. Between-staff communication can also present challenges; poor handover practices, differences in professional opinions, and a 'blame culture' were cited in this regard. These factors may be amplified in certain scenarios, e.g., when staffing levels are suboptimal, staff don't have a sophisticated understanding of dementia, the hospital culture is overly bureaucratic or change-resistant, and/or when staff are stressed or burning out.

One important enabler of person-centred care from the staff perspective was the presence of a dementia nurse specialist. Nurse specialists can educate other staff on making the physical environment more 'dementia-friendly', improve communication and relationships with patients/families, and support planning for a smoother, timelier discharge. Another enabler was the use of social and recreational activities which provide meaningful engagement for patients; however, the provision of the same was not always considered feasible.

The role of guidelines and self-assessment

Both the Irish (de Siún et al., 2014; Bracken-Scally et al., 2020) and the England and Wales (Royal College of Psychiatrists, 2019) dementia audits have reported incremental improvements in care policies and practices with each subsequent round, demonstrating the role of continuous monitoring and assessment for driving quality improvement. In this way, ongoing self-assessment by hospital staff might be a useful improvement strategy. One particularly influential and widely used ward environment assessment tool was developed by the King's Fund (2014), in collaboration with NHS trusts participating in the 'Enhancing the Healing Environment' (EHE) initiative. The EHE initiative was funded to support the implementation of the National Dementia Strategy in England. The tool was designed for single-user completion, however, the tool guidance emphasises the value of consulting multiple stakeholders (e.g., people with dementia, family members, and staff, including clinical, managerial, and estates personnel), to incorporate diverse views on the suitability of ward environments, and potential areas for improvement.

While evidence to support the effectiveness of dementia-friendly interventions is limited (Handley et al., 2017), Waller and Masterson (2015) have reported positive outcomes based on local data from 10 sites involved in the EHE initiative. The authors concluded that inexpensive, small-scale changes to the physical environment (e.g., using matte flooring, changing the colour of toilet doors) encouraged positive outcomes in relation to the prescribing of antipsychotic medication, and the incidence of aggression and falls. Making spaces seem less clinical, and reducing the number of decisions that must be made by patients in terms of wayfinding seems to significantly reduce agitation. Staff metrics also improved with reductions in absence rates and better recruitment and retention. Building and estates personnel reported that incorporating these design principles was not more costly than other similar-sized schemes.

Additionally, a multicentre retrospective cohort study by Kirch and Marquardt (2021) demonstrated that hospitalised patients (N = 2735) in specialist dementia wards with 'human-centred' designs, showed a significant improvement in self-care abilities post-discharge, i.e., mean Barthel Index scores increased from 35.3 (SD = 19.7) on admission, to 50.7 (SD = 24.9) at discharge. The use of the term 'human-centred' here reflects a call internationally to shift the focus of terminology from 'dementia-friendly' to 'universal design' principles (Grey et al., 2018). Advocates of this shift point out that hospitals cater for people of all ages with many conditions and diverse needs. Thus, the environment must be suitable for everyone. While making environments 'dementia friendly' may mean that they are universally suitable for all patients/visitors, the terminology may only appeal to those with a specific interest in championing dementia. Furthermore, hospital management and estates personnel have hospital-wide remits and thus are concerned with optimising hospital design for all. It is possible that the use of 'dementia-friendly' terminology, at least alone, might inherently imply to some stakeholders that the approach could inadvertently compromise the needs of other patient groups (though we don't believe this to be true). Instead, the term 'universal design' is inherently focused on making the environment accessible and easier to navigate for all patients and visitors, including those with dementia. Grey et al. (2018) published dementia design guidelines for hospital settings, incorporating a universal design approach. They make the case for guidelines being framed as 'dementia-supportive', rather than 'dementia-specific', and emphasise the role of universal design terminology in achieving this.

Conclusion

While there is substantial evidence pointing to the experiences and perspectives surrounding the organisation, provision, and receipt of hospital dementia care, and we understand some of the key deficits in the social and physical environment, more research is needed to ultimately improve experiences and outcomes. It is important that hospitals use self-assessment tools to evaluate their own ward environments, as such data gives clear indications for improvement in environmental design. While 'dementia-friendly' has become the popular framing of this issue, we may need more discussion regarding the suitability of this terminology in the context of hospital settings. There is a need for high-quality evidence on the effectiveness, sustainability, and cost-benefit of specific design characteristics in relation to the physical environment, to assist with service planning for changing population needs. Furthermore, a glaring omission in the existing body of literature relates to the lack of research incorporating a co-design approach to developing hospitals' social and physical environments, such that people with dementia, family members, and other often-excluded stakeholders (e.g., estates personnel) contribute to all stages of research processes in a meaningful way. Other potentially important considerations for future research include factors relating to climate change and pandemic-proofing.

In-depth box

- This chapter considers the role of the psychosocial and physical aspects of the hospital environment in dementia care.
- We synthesise data relating to outcomes; experiences of care recipients, family carers, and care providers; current care policies/practices; environmental interventions and quality improvement and audit initiatives.
- Additionally, we outline (1) the role of guidelines and hospital/ward self-evaluation; (2) the need for high-quality evidence on the effectiveness, sustainability, and cost-benefit of various design characteristics; and (3) the lack of co-designed hospital environment research which meaningfully includes people with dementia.
- Other important considerations for future research include factors relating to climate change and pandemic-proofing.

References

Ahmed, S., Leurent, B., & Sampson, E. L. (2014). Risk factors for incident delirium among older people in acute hospital medical units: A systematic review and meta-analysis. *Age and Ageing, 43*(3), 326–333.

Bracken-Scally, M., Timmons, S., O'Shea, E., Gallagher, P., Kennelly, S. P., Hamilton, V., & O Neill, D. (2020). *Report of the second Irish national audit of dementia care in acute hospitals*. The National Dementia Office.

Brady, N. M., Manning, E., O'Shea, E., O'Regan, N. A., Meagher, D., & Timmons, S. (2016). Hospital discharge data-sets grossly under-represent dementia-related activity in acute hospitals: A cohort study in five Irish acute hospitals. *International Journal of Geriatric Psychiatry, 31*(12), 1371–1372.

Briggs, R., Dyer, A., Nabeel, S., Collins, R., Doherty, J., Coughlan, T., O'neill, D., & Kennelly, S. (2017). Dementia in the acute hospital: The prevalence and clinical outcomes of acutely unwell patients with dementia. *QJM: An International Journal of Medicine, 110*(1), 33–37.

Brooker, D., & Latham, I. (2015). *Person-centred dementia care: Making services better with the VIPS framework*. Jessica Kingsley Publishers.

Burgstaller, M., Mayer, H., Schiess, C., & Saxer, S. (2018). Experiences and needs of relatives of people with dementia in acute hospitals—A meta-synthesis of qualitative studies. *Journal of Clinical Nursing, 27*(3–4), 502–515.

Carter, L., Yadav, A., O'Neill, S., & O'Shea, E. (2023). Extended length of stay and related costs associated with dementia in acute care hospitals in Ireland. *Aging & Mental Health, 27*(5), 911–920.

Chenoweth, L., Cook, J., & Williams, A. (2021). Perceptions of care quality during an acute hospital stay for persons with dementia and family/carers. *Healthcare (2227–9032), 9*(9), 1176–1190.

de Siún, A., O'Shea, E., Timmons, S., McArdle, D., Gibbons, P., O Neill, D., Kennelly, S. P., & Gallagher, P. (2014). *Irish national audit of dementia care in acute hospitals*. National Audit of Dementia Care.

Digby, R., & Bloomer, M. J. (2014). People with dementia and the hospital environment: The view of patients and family carers. *International Journal of Older People Nursing*, 9(1), 34–43.

Duah-Owusu White, M., & Kelly, F. (2023). A narrative review of staff views about dementia care in hospital through the lens of a systems framework. *Journal of Research in Nursing*, 28(2), 120–140.

Grey, T., Xidous, D., Kennelly, S., Mahon, S., Mannion, V., de Freine, P., Dockrell, D., de Siún, A., Murphy, N., & O'Neill, D. (2018). *Dementia friendly hospitals from a universal design approach-design guidelines 2018*. Dementia Services Information and Development Centre.

Gwernan-Jones, R., Abbott, R., Lourida, I., Rogers, M., Green, C., Ball, S., Hemsley, A., Cheeseman, D., Clare, L., & Moore, D. A. (2020). The experiences of hospital staff who provide care for people living with dementia: A systematic review and synthesis of qualitative studies. *International Journal of Older People Nursing*, 15(4), e12325.

Han, Q. Y. C., Rodrigues, N. G., Klainin-Yobas, P., Haugan, G., & Wu, X. V. (2022). Prevalence, risk factors, and impact of delirium on hospitalized older adults with dementia: A systematic review and meta-analysis. *Journal of the American Medical Directors Association*, 23(1), 23–32.

Handley, M., Bunn, F., & Goodman, C. (2017). Dementia-friendly interventions to improve the care of people living with dementia admitted to hospitals: A realist review. *BMJ Open*, 7(7), e015257.

Houghton, C., Murphy, K., Brooker, D., & Casey, D. (2016). Healthcare staffs' experiences and perceptions of caring for people with dementia in the acute setting: Qualitative evidence synthesis. *International Journal of Nursing Studies*, 61, 104–116.

Keuning-Plantinga, A., Roodbol, P., van Munster, B. C., & Finnema, E. J. (2021). Experiences of informal caregivers of people with dementia with nursing care in acute hospitals: A descriptive mixed-methods study. *Journal of Advanced Nursing*, 77(12), 4887–4899.

King's Fund. (2014). *Is your ward dementia friendly? EHE Environmental Assessment Tool*. The King's Fund.

Kirch, J., & Marquardt, G. (2021). Towards human-centred general hospitals: The potential of dementia-friendly design. *Architectural Science Review*, 66(5), 382–390.

Lehmann, J., Michalowsky, B., Kaczynski, A., Thyrian, J. R., Schenk, N. S., Esser, A., Zwingmann, I., & Hoffmann, W. (2018). The impact of hospitalization on readmission, institutionalization, and mortality of people with dementia: A systematic review and meta-analysis. *Journal of Alzheimer's Disease*, 64(3), 735–749.

Manietta, C., Purwins, D., Reinhard, A., Knecht, C., & Roes, M. (2022). Characteristics of dementia-friendly hospitals: An integrative review. *BMC Geriatrics*, 22(1), 1–16.

Morandi, A., Di Santo, S. G., Zambon, A., Mazzone, A., Cherubini, A., Mossello, E., Bo, M., Marengoni, A., Bianchetti, A., & Cappa, S. (2019). Delirium, dementia, and in-hospital mortality: The results from the Italian Delirium Day 2016, a national multicenter study. *The Journals of Gerontology: Series A*, 74(6), 910–916.

Nørgaard, A., Jensen-Dahm, C., Wimberley, T., Svendsen, J. H., Ishtiak-Ahmed, K., Laursen, T. M., Waldemar, G., & Gasse, C. (2022). Effect of antipsychotics on mortality risk in patients with dementia with and without comorbidities. *Journal of the American Geriatrics Society, 70*(4), 1169–1179.

Parke, B., Boltz, M., Hunter, K. F., Chambers, T., Wolf-Ostermann, K., Adi, M. N., Feldman, F., & Gutman, G. (2017). A scoping literature review of dementia-friendly hospital design. *The Gerontologist, 57*(4), e62–e74.

Parke, B., & Chappell, N. L. (2010). Transactions between older people and the hospital environment: A social ecological analysis. *Journal of Aging Studies, 24*(2), 115–124.

Pedone, C., Ercolani, S., Catani, M., Maggio, D., Ruggiero, C., Quartesan, R., Senin, U., Mecocci, P., & Cherubini, A. (2005). Elderly patients with cognitive impairment have a high risk for functional decline during hospitalization: The GIFA Study. *The Journals of Gerontology Series A: Biological Sciences and Medical Sciences, 60*(12), 1576–1580.

Prince, M., Comas-Herrera, A., Knapp, M., Guerchet, M., & Karagiannidou, M. (2016). *World Alzheimer report 2016: Improving healthcare for people living with dementia: Coverage, quality and costs now and in the future.* Alzheimer Disease International.

Rao, A., Suliman, A., Vuik, S., Aylin, P., & Darzi, A. (2016). Outcomes of dementia: Systematic review and meta-analysis of hospital administrative database studies. *Archives of Gerontology and Geriatrics, 66,* 198–204.

Reilly, J. C., & Houghton, C. (2019). The experiences and perceptions of care in acute settings for patients living with dementia: A qualitative evidence synthesis. *International Journal of Nursing Studies, 96,* 82–90.

Reynish, E., Hapca, S., Walesby, R., Pusram, A., Bu, F., Burton, J. K., Cvoro, V., Galloway, J., Ebbesen Laidlaw, H., & Latimer, M. (2021). Understanding health-care outcomes of older people with cognitive impairment and/or dementia admitted to hospital: A mixed-methods study. *Health Services and Delivery Research, 9*(8), 1–280.

Reynish, E., Hapca, S. M., De Souza, N., Cvoro, V., Donnan, P. T., & Guthrie, B. (2017). Epidemiology and outcomes of people with dementia, delirium, and unspecified cognitive impairment in the general hospital: Prospective cohort study of 10,014 admissions. *BMC Medicine, 15*(1), 1–12.

Royal College of Psychiatrists. (2011). *Report of the National Audit of Dementia Care in General Hospitals.* Healthcare Quality Improvement Partnership.

Royal College of Psychiatrists. (2019). *National audit of dementia care in general hospitals 2018–19: Round four audit report.* Healthcare Quality Improvement Partnership.

Scerri, A., Scerri, C., & Innes, A. (2020). The perceived and observed needs of patients with dementia admitted to acute medical wards. *Dementia, 19*(6), 1997–2017.

Timmons, S., Bracken-Scally, M., Chakraborty, S., Gallagher, P., Hamilton, V., Begley, E., & O'Shea, E. (2023). Psychotropic medication prescribing to patients with dementia admitted to acute hospitals in Ireland. *Drugs & Aging, 40*(5), 461–472.

Timmons, S., Manning, E., Barrett, A., Brady, N. M., Browne, V., O'Shea, E., Molloy, D. W., O'Regan, N. A., Trawley, S., & Cahill, S. (2015). Dementia in older people admitted to hospital: A regional multi-hospital observational study of prevalence, associations and case recognition. *Age and Ageing, 44*(6), 993–999.

Toot, S., Devine, M., Akporobaro, A., & Orrell, M. (2013). Causes of hospital admission for people with dementia: A systematic review and meta-analysis. *Journal of the American Medical Directors Association*, 14(7), 463–470.

Topo, P., Kotilainen, H., & Eloniemi-Sulkava, U. (2012). Affordances of the care environment for people with dementia—An assessment study. *HERD: Health Environments Research & Design Journal*, 5(4), 118–138.

Turner, A., Eccles, F. J., Elvish, R., Simpson, J., & Keady, J. (2017). The experience of caring for patients with dementia within a general hospital setting: A meta-synthesis of the qualitative literature. *Aging & Mental Health*, 21(1), 66–76.

Waller, S., & Masterson, A. (2015). Designing dementia-friendly hospital environments. *Future Hospital Journal*, 2(1), 63–68.

Architectural design guidance for general hospitals

Ways to implement proven concepts and to accommodate future challenges

Gesine Marquardt and Kathrin Bueter

Hospitalization of people with dementia as a complex challenge

Our aging societies are contributing to a growing population of older adults requiring hospital care. Around 40 percent of patients aged over 65 display cognitive impairments, and approximately one-fifth exhibit symptoms of dementia (Hendlmeier et al., 2018). Yet dementia is seldom the primary reason for hospitalization.

Even when dementia is diagnosed, it tends to be secondary, despite its potential to significantly influence treatment outcomes and therapeutic processes. More commonly, hospitalizations result from falls, fractures, malnutrition, cardiac, respiratory, gastrointestinal ailments, infections, and behavioural challenges. Often, patients grapple with multiple coexisting conditions (Rao et al., 2016). Yet, the complex interplay of social factors also plays a role in the hospitalization equation: Individuals living with dementia experience higher hospitalization rates, but their requirements lean more towards caregiving and supervision, and they receive therapeutic or diagnostic treatment at a lower rate than persons of the same age who do not have symptoms of dementia. Still, costs of hospital treatment for people with dementia were found to be higher than their peers (Motzek et al., 2018).

Older patients with dementia often display behaviours that constitute a challenge to the established hospital processes that predominantly cater to patients who comprehend the purpose of their hospitalization and who are willing to cooperate with their treatments. As people with dementia disrupt the rigid clinical protocols, it may lead to the perception of these patients as a disruption to the smooth functioning of the hospital's operations (Bail et al., 2015). At the same time that patient numbers are rising, hospitals confront significant challenges with staff shortages. Fewer nurses must now manage more patients in less time, while also addressing the distinctive and time-intensive support requirements of dementia patients.

Finally, hospitalization is a major challenge to the people with dementia themselves. The German Alzheimer's Society describes hospital stays for

DOI: 10.4324/9781003416241-17

dementia patients as "one of the most difficult situations to deal with in their condition" (Deutsche Alzheimer Gesellschaft, 2013). Uprooted from their familiar surroundings, hospitalization becomes a crisis for these individuals. The shift in location, unfamiliar routines, and absence of familiar faces lead to anxiety, insecurity, and disorientation. Many struggle to articulate these challenges and instead respond with intense emotions like fear, unease, aggression, or withdrawal. Further, they face a higher risk of falls, delirium, and post-operative complications during their stay. Cognitive decline often sets in, erasing familiarity with daily tasks. Consequently, discharge to the home environment becomes unfeasible, leading to transfers to nursing homes.

Architectural Design to address hospitalization challenges

Patients should be the focus of all design considerations in the hospital and the design of their spatial environment should positively influence their experience and recovery. At the same time, hospitals are also central hubs where medical and nursing workflows take place, so the design must also facilitate optimum performance of these processes. Additional parameters influencing architectural design include economic factors and the fulfilment of medical, technical, and hygienic requirements. Balancing these diverse criteria requires seamless integration within a comprehensive overall concept. Dementia-friendly design needs to be an integral part of this concept. This implies that the architectural design of hospitals aims to counteract compromised coping skills by creating environments that enhance well-being, orientation, safety, and the ability to sustain self-care routines. Extensive reviews of existing literature support this correlation within nursing home settings (Calkins, 2018; Chaudhury et al., 2018; Fleming, Zeisel, and Bennett, 2020a).

While a significant portion of the available research originates from nursing home settings, design approaches can be extrapolated and tailored for implementation in general hospitals. Bueter and Marquardt (2021) have identified ten principles of dementia-sensitive architecture, encompassing guidance on: *1. the floor plan structure, 2. floor space requirements, 3. safety, 4. orientation, 5. guidance and orientation systems, 6. lighting, 7. colours and contrasts, 8. atmosphere, 9. activation concepts,* and 10. *stimulus densities.* With these guiding principles in mind, architectural design concepts for dementia-friendly environments within hospital settings can be developed. And indeed, over the past decade, there has been a growing movement towards implementing dementia-friendly design in hospital facilities, resulting in the publication of case studies and design recommendations (The Kings Fund, 2017; Fleming, Zeisel, and Bennett, 2020b; Bueter and Marquardt, 2021). Even the efficacy in preserving critical self-care capabilities of patients with dementia through specific design measures has been demonstrated (Kirch and Marquardt, 2021). Examining the design approaches available clarifies that dementia-friendly design strategies aim to enhance the built environment's clarity and attentiveness to human requirements. While patients with dementia may be particularly sensitive to their surroundings, it's important to acknowledge that all individuals being treated as hospital patients are vulnerable. Thus, a supportive design benefits everyone in this context.

Key architectural design recommendations for hospitals

We conducted a series of research and design projects in various hospital settings. Our tasks included analysing existing dementia-friendly hospital wards, consulting with architects and healthcare providers who were at the time involved in the construction of new hospital buildings and implementing two original architectural designs (one for a hospital ward and another for an emergency department, as detailed in Bueter and Marquardt, 2021). Our architectural design projects were consistently accompanied by research efforts. Individuals with dementia participated in these projects. In one instance, we extensively documented their spatial behaviours within the ward before and after remodelling. In another, we asked for their opinions on the interior design of rooms. In yet another project, we distributed questionnaires to proxies (caregivers and healthcare professionals) to gather their input. Furthermore, representatives from patient self-help organizations participated in workshops and provided valuable feedback on our work.

As an outcome of our research and design efforts for almost a decade, we have identified three crucial aspects within the hospital setting that significantly affect the hospital stay of individuals with dementia: (i) the seamless integration of the hospital structure into its urban surroundings, (ii) the incorporation of dementia-friendly elements in the emergency department, and (iii) the establishment of spatial anchor points within hospital wards (Bueter and Marquardt, 2021).

Integrate hospitals into urban environments

Hospitals, previously destinations solely for illness, are now evolving into centres for comprehensive well-being. Their design should embrace this transformation by shifting away from isolated structures on enclosed campuses, and instead, integrate seamlessly within urban landscapes. This helps people with dementia to have a less disruptive transfer into the new environment as it looks similar to what they know, allowing them to employ their established orientation strategies.

Expand the City Fabric: Hospitals must become integral to urban development, with pathways linking the hospital campus to public spaces. Open-plan spaces with services like cafes and events enhance the community's quality of life. Design coherence with the surroundings is vital, aiding familiar navigation especially for people with dementia. By weaving hospitals into daily urban routes, anxieties linked to hospitalization can diminish.

Design a Micro-Cosmos: Beyond core medical functions, hospitals encompass diverse amenities. Adhering solely to building regulations can lead to complex, disorienting layouts. Hospitals should emulate urban networks, forming nodes for social interaction and tranquillity. Urban concepts, like a hospital "aorta" with varying interconnected spaces, guide the building's structure and can be extended to medical areas.

Facilitate Orientation: The main strategy is to create spatial situations that are legible, memorable, and thus recognizable in function and meaning, with a structure and design that permits individuals living with dementia to use familiar orientational and behavioural strategies. Familiar spatial cues aid navigation for patients with dementia. At the same time, the inclusion of individuals with sensory impairment needs to be addressed through the provision of multi-sensory navigation aids.

Enhance Recreation: Tranquil spots with high recreational value are crucial, especially in bustling hospitals. Amidst sensory stimuli, patients need moments of respite. Shielded areas in circulation zones or cafeterias provide solace. Controlled stimuli, referencing nature or activities, replace overwhelming distractions.

Provide Accessible Information: Clear guidance is imperative in complex hospitals. Central information hubs, manned by approachable staff, offer vital assistance. Visual distinction, varied counter heights, and privacy considerations ensure inclusivity and accessibility (Figure 12.1).

Meet varied requirements in dementia-friendly emergency departments

Creating dementia-friendly emergency departments presents a distinct challenge. These spaces are primarily designed for intense functionality and optimized workflows, prioritizing medical requirements and staff needs. Patient needs frequently assume a secondary role. However, these departments serve as crucial entry points for individuals living with dementia who frequently require emergency care. This initial interaction significantly influences subsequent care and outcomes, particularly considering higher mortality rates, decreased self-reliance, and elevated delirium risk among elderly patients attending emergency departments. This underscores the pressing necessity for a tailored care structure and design that is responsive to dementia-related needs.

Shield the Waiting Area: Presenting in an emergency department often involves long, strenuous waits. Design projects have shown the benefits of a dedicated waiting area for patients living with dementia and their family members. A dementia-friendly waiting area is a distinct, quiet, and shielded area, separate from its surroundings, and offers protection from the hustle and bustle, noise, and occasionally disturbing happenings in an emergency department.

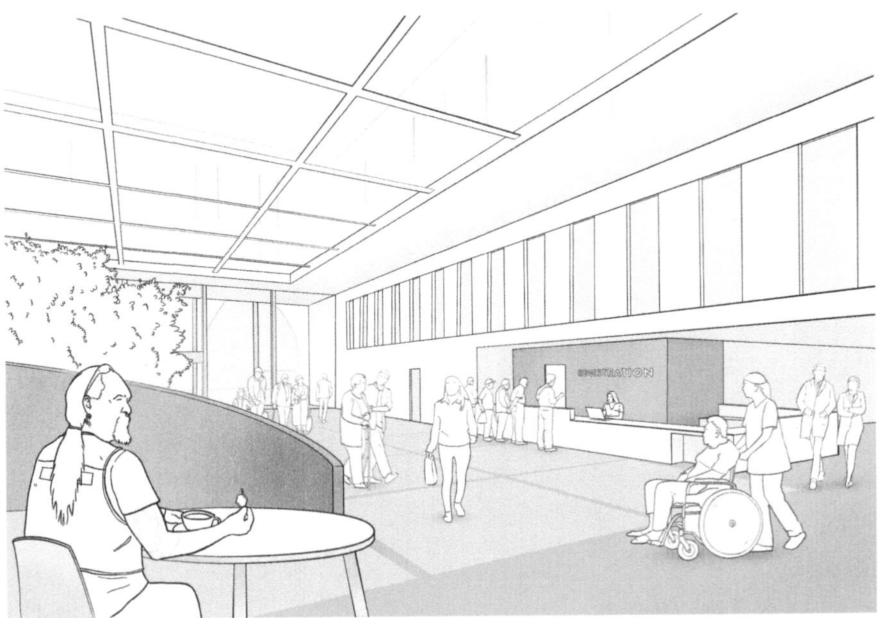

Figure 12.1 Central hall of a hospital where aspects of urban life are reflected. Clear lines of sight from seating area to the registration desk provide orientation and a sense of security.

Source: Bueter and Marquardt, 2021.

Older patients can wait there with family members or companions, as they can calm the patients and given them a sense of security. Patients and relatives can maintain eye contact with a specific contact person. That gives both parties a sense of security and control. Seating and reclining spaces provide reprieve, while the waiting time can also be utilized for activities, aided by ample room for movement and engaging diversions. An appealing outside view can serve as a welcomed distraction. Nearby amenities, such as a unisex accessible restroom, refreshments suited to the patient group, are conveniently accessible.

Adapt Examination and Treatment Rooms: Patients are always accompanied by medical staff to the diagnostic and treatment areas in an emergency department. In areas like shock and procedure rooms, process-optimized design must be prioritized. However, in order to cater to the needs of patients with dementia, a key goal is to allow family members or other caregivers to accompany them. Their presence not only gives people with dementia a sense of security, but they also communicate for the patients when necessary, assist with describing symptoms and conditions, and take in information on further necessary treatments. There must be enough space to allow caregivers to be close to the patients with movable, comfortable seating. If treatment is required, they should be able to withdraw within the room. At the same

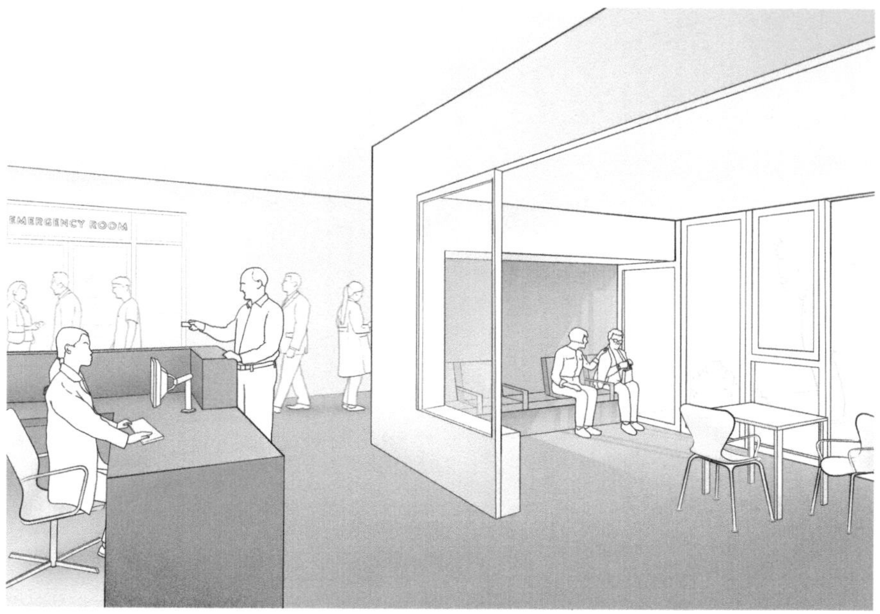

Figure 12.2 Within the emergency room, a secluded waiting area designed for patients with dementia and their relatives is situated near the central nursing desk. The provision of outward views offers a source of distraction, and ample space is available for unrestricted movement.

Source: Bueter and Marquardt, 2021.

time, in treatment rooms key design approaches for dementia-friendly design should be implemented, such as good acoustics to make it easier to follow communication or interior design elements like (day-) light, colours, pictures, and views can distract and calm patients (Figure 12.2).

Provide spatial anchor points in the wards

Specialized wards exclusively admitting individuals with dementia have proven advantageous in delivering care for those patients. Nonetheless, the majority of general hospitals lack such specialized units. Consequently, individuals with dementia can be encountered across various departments, underscoring the need to enhance the dementia-friendliness of standard wards. Therefore, each hospital ward should incorporate a spatial anchor point, a crucial landmark aiding patient navigation. A space qualifies as such if it possesses distinct spatial attributes, high visibility, and effortless accessibility. The area is also lively, offering patient interaction and engagement. People with dementia often seek companionship, making the presence of others a pivotal orientation element alongside the spatial arrangement and design of the area.

Position the Spatial Anchor Point: The importance of the spatial anchor point's placement within the ward cannot be overstated, as its location significantly influences patients' activity. One approach is to cluster the nursing station, communal space, and entrance in proximity to each other. This arrangement offers clear sightlines between the entrance and nursing station, providing an immediate point of contact upon entering the ward. Conversely, an exposed exit might inadvertently facilitate patients' unnoticed departure. Alternatively, positioning the spatial anchor point at the ward's core, with the entrance farther away and less visually engaging, discourages patient exploration and self-exit. Yet, this approach lacks the advantage of immediate contact with staff upon entry. Regardless of the chosen layout, effective signage guiding patients intuitively to the spatial anchor point is particularly important.

Equip the Spatial Anchor Point: To encourage patient interaction and engagement, specific elements are crucial. Foremost, adequate seating arrangements are essential, catering to conversational interactions among patients, visitors, and staff, as well as providing tranquil spaces for observation. These seating options should facilitate effortless communication between patients and offer private viewpoints when needed. Notably, the ability to observe the staff holds particular significance, as it enhances patients' feelings of security. To promote staff accessibility, considering the inclusion of a reception counter at the spatial anchor point is advantageous. This counter should possess clear visibility, inviting aesthetics, and convey the approachability of the nursing staff. The design should facilitate eye-level communication, achieved through varying counter heights that accommodate both seated and standing interactions. Ensuring continuous staffing is vital as an unattended counter might inadvertently create a sense of unease. Therefore, if adequate staffing cannot be maintained, it may be preferable to omit the counter. In addition to facilitating communication and observation, the spatial anchor point should provide patients with engaging activities. Offering diversions like photobooks, magazines, and headphones for storytelling or music can provide sources of entertainment. Furthermore, recognizing the concern of malnutrition among older adults, easy access to beverages and light snacks should be readily available. Finally, an accessible bathroom should also be in the line of sight from the seating area of the spatial anchor point (Figure 12.3).

Directions for future hospital designs

Dementia-friendly design can be effectively implemented while adhering to the multitude of regulations and requirements prevalent in healthcare environments. The highlighted key architectural design recommendations underscore that innovative architectural solutions addressing the needs of individuals with dementia can also be successfully integrated into retrofit situations.

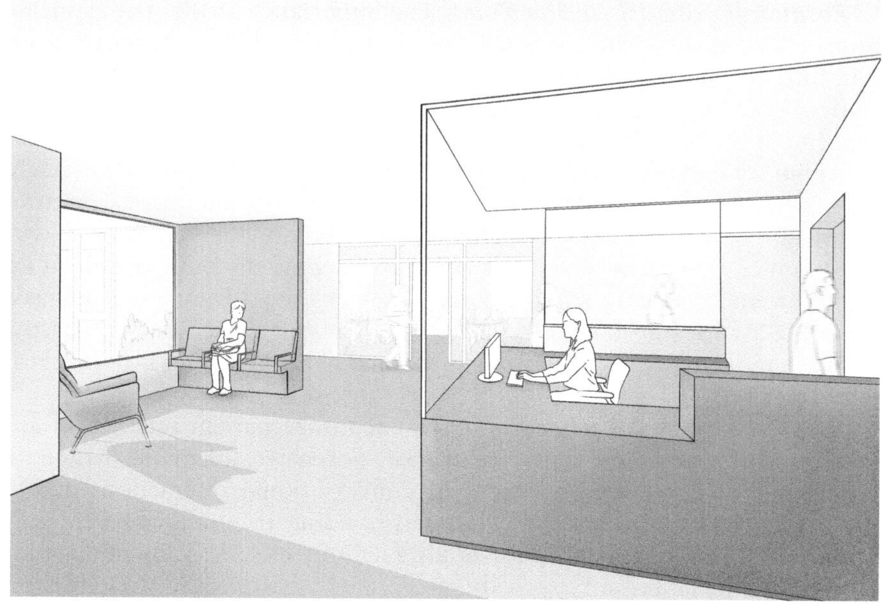

Figure 12.3 A central space within the hospital ward serves as a spatial anchor for patients, allowing them to sit, engage with others, observe the staff, or simply enjoy views of the surroundings.

Source: Bueter and Marquardt, 2021.

Still, it is necessary to decide on how to incorporate the needs of the ageing population and the increasing numbers of patients living with dementia as early as in the requirement planning state of a project. All future participants must be considered in the planning process and after the building is commissioned, action must be taken to ensure that it is used in accordance with the defined goals. In existing hospital buildings, a systematic evaluation can identify potential for readjustment.

When undertaking the planning of hospital buildings, architects and healthcare providers should refrain from relying solely on insights drawn from past projects. This is particularly crucial when the designs are not grounded in systematic research evidence. Even when integrating research findings, there are inherent challenges to contend with. Not all decisions pertaining to architectural design can be fully substantiated by existing research, since the scope of architectural evidence to support design decisions remains constrained. Conflicting requirements often arise, necessitating a harmonization process, especially in relation to intended nursing procedures, workflow arrangements, and financial considerations for construction budgets and ongoing maintenance costs of the hospital buildings.

Further, the research available stems from sources that researchers around the globe were pushing forward. While there are many similarities between hospital designs in many countries, it is imperative to also consider cultural values and expectations. In cases involving individuals with dementia, their inclusion during the planning phase becomes paramount. Factors such as furnishings, colour selections, and related elements demand their input. Participatory approaches, encompassing models, prototypes, and mood boards, can effectively capture their design preferences (Branco, Quental, and Ribeiro, 2017).

Lastly, apprehensions often arise surrounding the creation of dementia-friendly healthcare facilities, notably from the perspective of healthcare providers. There is concern that such an emphasis might lead to a stigmatized perception of the establishment, potentially dissuading other user groups. This predicament can be mitigated by seamlessly infusing dementia-friendly design principles into the architecture, achieving a synthesis within the overall concept. This inclusive approach not only averts immediate discernibility but also contributes to elevating the architectural design quality of the entire hospital building.

Conclusion

The growing body of research on dementia-sensitive design can be a driver for innovative hospital design that caters to the needs of all user groups, thus paving the way for a human-centred hospital design. The key architectural design recommendations highlighted in this chapter are highly specific to the needs of people with dementia during their hospital stay, but at the same time can be implemented in a non-stigmatizing way and thus be beneficial for all patients. Moreover, individuals who are vulnerable, such as people with dementia, tend to be acutely attuned to their surroundings, amplifying their fundamental human requirements. Directing greater attention towards these individuals and their needs could heighten architects' sensitivity, as they can be indicators of the environment's design quality. Their perceived vulnerability might even be re-envisioned as a strength, as it offers designers clearer insights into how the environment affects its user. Ultimately, all individuals share common essential needs: serenity, purpose, safety, direction, positive engagement, and social interaction – requisites frequently overlooked in healthcare settings. Incorporating these notions into architectural design offers a reliable pathway to cultivating a more empathetic architecture, specifically customized to cater to the needs of all individuals. Consequently, improved healthcare outcomes can be anticipated, with research even suggesting a potential link between well-designed architecture and increased staff satisfaction, coupled with reduced staff turnover – vital considerations in the context of demographic shifts.

In-depth box

- Dementia-friendly designs within general hospitals yield favourable effects on the well-being of individuals with dementia, extending to positive outcomes for staff members as well.
- Feasibility is a notable aspect of integrating dementia-friendly design within general hospitals, applicable to both newly constructed and renovated structures.
- The adoption of dementia-friendly design principles in general hospitals promotes inclusivity across diverse user groups.
- Dementia-friendly design can be seamlessly integrated to enhance aesthetics and overall architectural quality of hospital buildings.

Acknowledgements

We gratefully acknowledge the support of the Robert Bosch Stiftung Stuttgart, Germany, for their generous funding, which has played an instrumental role in enabling the realization of our research and design projects on hospital design al for people with dementia.

References

Bail, K., Goss, J., Draper, B., Berry, H., Karmel, R., & Gibson, D. (2015). The Cost of Hospital-Acquired Complications for Older People with and Without Dementia; a Retrospective Cohort Study. *BMCHealth Services Research* 15 (March): 91. doi:10.1186/s12913-015-0743-1.

Branco, R. M., Quental, J., & Ribeiro, Ó. (2017). Personalised Participation: An Approach to Involve People with Dementia and their Families in a Participatory Design Project. *CoDesign*, 13 (2): 127–143.

Bueter, K., & Marquardt, G. (2021). *Dementia-friendly Hospital Buildings. Construction and Design Manual*. Berlin: DOM Publishing.

Calkins, M. P. (2018). From Research to Application: Supportive and Therapeutic Environments for People Living with Dementia. *The Gerontologist* 58 (Suppl_1): S114–S128. doi:10.1093/geront/gnx146.

Chaudhury, H., Cooke, H. A., Cowie, H., & Razaghi, L. (2018) The Influence of the Physical Environment on Residents with Dementia in Long-term Care Settings: A Review of the Empirical Literature. *The Gerontologist* 58 (5): e325–e337. doi:10.1093/geront/gnw259.

Deutsche Alzheimer Gesellschaft (Hrsg.) (2013). *Menschen mit Demenz im Krankenhaus. Auf dem Weg zum demenzsensiblen Krankenhaus*. Berlin: Deutsche Alzheimer Gesellschaft e.V.

Fleming, R., Zeisel, J., & Bennett, K. (2020a). *World Alzheimer Report 2020: Design Dignity Dementia: Dementia-related Design and the Built Environment, Volume 1*. Alzheimer's Disease International. https://www.alzint.org/u/WorldAlzheimerReport2020Vol1.pdf

Fleming, R., Zeisel, J., & Bennett, K. (2020b). *World Alzheimer Report 2020: Design Dignity Dementia: Dementia-related Design and the Built Environment, Volume 2*. Alzheimer's Disease International. https://www.alzint.org/u/WorldAlzheimerReport2020Vol2.pdf

Hendlmeier, I., Bickel, H., Hessler, J. B., Weber, J., Junge, M. N., Leonhardt, S., & Schäufele, M. (2018). Dementia Friendly Care Services in General Hospitals: Representative Results of the General Hospital Study (GHoSt). *Zeitschrift für Gerontologie und Geriatrie*, 51:509–516.

The King's Fund (2017) Environments of Care for People with Dementia. https://www.kingsfund.org.uk/projects/enhancing-healing-environment/completed-projects

Kirch, J., & Marquardt, G. (2021). Towards Human-centred General Hospitals: The Potential of Dementia-friendly Design. *Architectural Science Review*, 66 (5): 382–390.

Motzek, T., Werblow, A., Tesch, F., Marquardt, G., & Schmitt, J. (2018). Determinants of Hospitalization and Length of Stay among People with Dementia–An Analysis of Statutory Health Insurance Claims Data. *Archives of Gerontology and Geriatrics*, 76:227–233.

Rao, A., A. Suliman, S. Vuik, P. Aylin, & A. Darzi. 2016. Outcomes of Dementia: Systematic Review and Meta-analysis of Hospital Administrative Database Studies. *Archives of Gerontology and Geriatrics* 66 (September): 198–204. doi:10.1016/j.archger.2016.06.008.

Care home design

Translating environmental design knowledge into practice

Progress and challenges

Richard Fleming and John Zeisel

This article is based on the professional experience of the two authors on opposite sides of the globe living and working in the decades during which evidence-based dementia-specific knowledge has moved through the four stages of awareness, agreement, adoption, and adherence.

"Virtually every country in the world is experiencing growth in the size and proportion of older people in their population" (United Nations, 2019). With the incidence of dementia highly correlated with age, this means a greater incidence of dementia in all countries. While older adults express a desire to stay in their own homes as they age, many become frail, develop chronic and complex diseases, and require long-term residential care in the final stages of their life (Hatcher et al., 2019).

Evidence-based psycho-social interventions improve the well-being and daily life of residents with dementia in long-term care settings (Zeisel, 2010). Environmental interventions (Charras et al., 2016; Chaudhury et al., 2017; Fleming & Purandare, 2010; Zeisel et al., 2016) also contribute in a major way (Fleming et al., 2016). While there are many examples of dementia design knowledge incorporated in buildings-in-use, the regulatory application of this knowledge is weak, as evidenced by the lack of reference to environmental interventions in National Dementia Plans (Golembiewski, 2020).

The gap between research knowledge and its application in regulations is well known with numerous explanations proposed for this gap (Draper et al., 2009).

A conceptual model featuring four stages of moving new knowledge into practice has been proposed by Pathman (Pathman et al., 1996).

1 Raising *awareness* of new knowledge
2 Gaining *agreement* that the new knowledge requires a change in practice and agreeing to participate in that change
3 *Adoption* of the new knowledge in practice
4 *Adherence* with the new knowledge and associated practices realised as part of business as usual, often supported by guidelines and/or regulations [(Pathman et al., 1996, p. 873].

DOI: 10.4324/9781003416241-19

Emergence of a set of design principles

Since the 1980s, there have been several attempts to define good design for people living with dementia, with successive sets of design criteria mirroring the others. In an early Australian paper Fleming (Fleming & Bowles, 1987) identified eight principles of good design: small size; provision of domestic facilities; easy access to local community; reduction of unhelpful stimulation; highlighting of helpful stimuli; good visual access – that is, residents able to see where they want to go; provision of opportunities for social interaction; and maintaining familiar surroundings through familiar furniture, fittings, and décor.

In the following decade in the US, several social scientists and architectural researchers approached the same taxonomic task. Cohen and Weisman (1991) described nine goals for the environment: ensure safety and security; support functional ability through meaningful activity; maximise awareness and orientation; provide opportunities for stimulation and change; maximise autonomy and control; adapt to changing needs; establish links to the healthy and familiar; provide opportunities for socialisation; and protect privacy.

Comparing and summarising the work of Cohen and Weisman together with the ground-breaking analysis of Lawton (Lawton, 1990) and Calkins (Calkins, 1988) Zeisel et al., proposed an environment-behaviour (E-B) model for Alzheimer special care units with eight primary environmental characteristics: exit control; wandering paths; individual away places; common space structure; outdoor freedom; residential scale; autonomy support; and sensory comprehension (Zeisel et al., 1994).

A decade later in Scotland Marshall (Marshall, 2001) promoted facility design that are small in size; domestic and homelike; provide scope for ordinary activities (unit kitchens, washing lines, garden sheds); have unobtrusive safety features; have rooms for different functions, with furniture and fittings familiar to the age and generation of the residents; have a safe outside space; have single rooms big enough for a reasonable amount of personal belongings; have good signage and multiple cues where possible; use objects rather than colour for orientation; enhance visual access; and control stimuli, especially noise.

In 2003 Fleming in collaboration with Bennett (Fleming et al., 2003) expanded the 1987 principles to include unobtrusive safety measures and the principle of ensuring that buildings are designed with a clearly stated vision for a way of life of residents.

That these principles are common to the work of most well-known designers was tested by systematically sampling 443 books on design for dementia and 409 articles referenced by five major systematic reviews. After this rigorous analysis to assess agreement between the principles and the writings of international experts, Bennett, Fleming, and Zeisel (Bennett et al., 2020), employed them as the organising system for both data collection and presentation in the Alzheimer's Disease International's 2020 World Alzheimer Report, which includes contributions from 58 experts in 17 countries and, in Volume 2, 84 building case studies from 27 countries (Fleming et al., 2020). While the comparative analysis demonstrated great variety in terminology and how ideas were described, it showed broad agreement about what makes a good environment for people living with dementia, with the built-environment case studies all reflecting the principles.

The utility of the 2020 principles as a summary of existing knowledge was further demonstrated in responses to the online publication of the Dignity Manifesto for Design for people living with dementia (Fleming et al., 2021), published with an invitation for signatories to indicate agreement. As of the writing of this chapter, the online Design Dignity Manifesto has been signed by over 430 design professionals, academic researchers, policymakers, and people living with dementia.

The Dignity Manifesto principles are as follows:

- Begin each project by developing a vision for a dignified way of life for people living with dementia.
- Where safety measures are agreed to be appropriate, design them to be as unobtrusive as possible.
- Design the environment to reflect a human scale.
- Plan the environment to make it easy for people to see and move where they want to go.
- Optimise stimulation.
- Promote movement, engagement, and meaningfulness.
- Afford people opportunities to enjoy contact with nature
- Design all components of the environment to be as familiar as possible.
- Afford people opportunities to choose to be alone or with various size groups of people.
- Provide easy access and connection to and from local communities, families, and friends.

These consensus principles ("the Principles") represent a strong starting point for designing well for people living with dementia.

Stage one: awareness

Raising awareness is the critical first stage in introducing new ideas to practitioners and the public. One traditional method to raise awareness is publishing academic articles, with literature reviews often employed to establish new concepts and familiarise oneself with a field (Fleming & Purandare, 2010). Since literature reviews can be written without the need for fieldwork, this method is accessible to authors without the requirement of a grant.

The authors also raised awareness of new ideas by starting new journals. As early as 1970, Zeisel together with editor Ann Ferebee established Design & Environment, a professional journal to bridge the gap between psychological and social research knowledge and design.

In 2012, Fleming launched the Australian Journal of Dementia Care to showcase good practices and keep readers up to date on developments in dementia care practice. (https://journalofdementiacare.com/about/). This journal adopted the successful formula of The Journal of Dementia Care, established in 1993 by Dr. Richard Hawkins in the UK. The AJDC became a principal tool of knowledge translation in the Wollongong University-based Dementia Training Australia, established to provide dementia training to the aged care workforce with funding from the Australian Government (https://dta.com.au/). Environmental design was an area of particular interest to the AJDC founder, and many articles were dedicated to how the built environment could be leveraged to provide better care.

Massive Open Online Courses (MOOCs) have also proven successful in introducing large numbers of people to new ideas. The University of Tasmania has included a module on dementia-inclusive design in its MOOC since 2013, based on the extant principles (Fleming et al., 2003), with over 200,000 people enrolled in this MOOC (Farrow et al., 2018). The course has generated interest in the principles among people from countries as diverse as New Zealand and Ukraine. Similarly, Zeisel with medical colleagues Joel Belmin and Olivier Drunat established in 2010 an Inter-University Diploma Course on non-pharmacological treatment of dementia at the Sorbonne in Paris that includes a major component on the role of environmental design. While only hundreds of students have benefited in-person, the related MOOC has reached 24,503 international participants, from 90 countries.

Stage two: agreement

Agreement that incorporating specific new knowledge improves practice, requires that practitioners engage with and test the relevance to their practice of the knowledge, making it more difficult to achieve than raising awareness. Awareness requires attention; agreement requires action.

In the 1970s, courses in user needs of elders living with dementia were established in many architecture schools. Zeisel with colleague's architect Marc Maxwell, landscape architect David Kamp, Doctor Bill Thomas, and architectural researcher Victor Regnier taught a course on user needs in Assisted Living with an emphasis on design for dementia to practicing architects in the Harvard University Graduate School of Design Executive Education Program. Attended by major architectural firms involved with designing Memory Care Assisted Living Communities, some began immediately to apply these lessons. Among these was the architecture firm establishing prototypes of buildings developed and managed by Sunrise

Senior Living, an innovative large provider of residential dementia care at that time.

Between 2013 and 2016, Fleming worked with twelve schools in seven universities to deliver design studios to undergraduate students. All design studios began with an introduction to the role of the built environment in creating enabling environments where people living with dementia can be at their best. From there the studios developed in different ways depending on their context (Marcello et al., 2015). The Royal Melbourne Institute of Technology (RMIT University) adopted one of the most sophisticated approaches, describing the project:

> There is immense potential in the Dementia Project to enhance the student experience through a cross-disciplinary, industry engaged, design studio that assists to generate conceptual and practical solutions of relevance to the complex world of dementia.
>
> (Blythe & Nazareth, 2017)

A link to the book that came from RMIT's series of studios is included in the references.

The development of the Design Dignity Manifesto described earlier is a prime example of a conscious effort to increase not only awareness but also agreement with the principles. The action of signing the manifesto clearly signifies agreement and lays the foundation for the next stage, adoption.

Stage three: adoption

Adopting new knowledge among practitioners requires extensive engagement between knowledge providers and those practitioners who apply that new knowledge. Zeisel's Inquiry by Design (Zeisel, 1984, 2006) describes how developing new knowledge and developing architectural responses are similar creative processes with different emphases, naturally linked together.

The Environmental Design Service that Dementia Training Australia provides, exemplifies new knowledge adoption (https://dta.com.au/dementia-friendly-environments/). The service provides on-site education on the application of the principles in design and an assessment of the strengths and weaknesses of each designed facility using the Environmental Audit Tool (Fleming, 2011; Fleming & Bennett, 2015; Fleming & Bennett, 2019). This assessment provides the foundation for discussion of the design project. Graphing the results of the environmental audit reveals strengths and weaknesses of the design.

Figure 13.1 reflects a case study in which the greatest design concerns were the following principles: 'Provide a human scale', 'Familiarity', and 'Provide opportunities for engagement with ordinary life'. On the other hand, the case study facility responds well to the principles 'Optimise helpful stimulation' and 'Links to the community'.

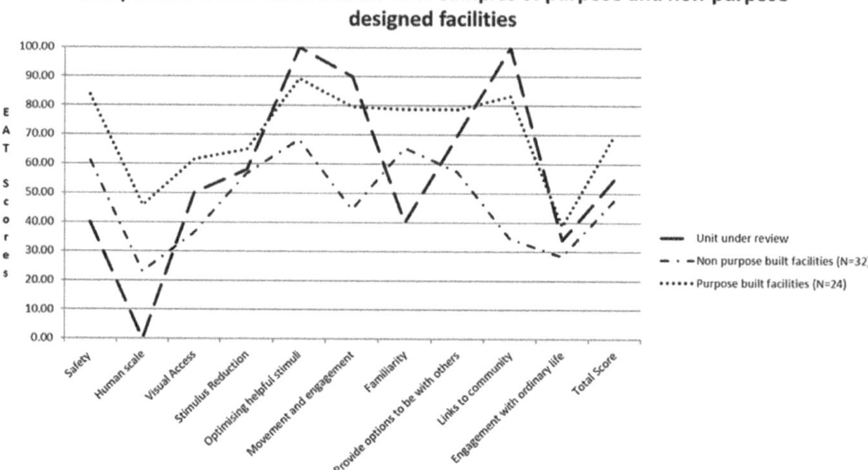

Figure 13.1 Environmental audit tool results for residential aged care facility.

Providing practitioners with tools that help them apply the principles themselves, effectively promotes adoption, yet is less intensive. The *Built Environment Audit Tool-Dementia* (BEAT-D) smart phone app, available from app stores, provides practitioners with a way to complete the Environmental Audit Tool themselves and receive a detailed report of the strengths and weaknesses of the building they are assessing.

PLAN-EAT (Quirke et al., 2023), another self-applied tool, can be used to assess residential aged care facilities floorplans, enabling practitioners to apply knowledge of the principles as they design. Employing PLAN-EAT architects are able to avoid problems that often become apparent only during post-occupancy evaluations.

Tools like these effectively shorten the journey from agreement to adoption.

Adoption by design in practice, i.e. constructed buildings in use – serve as concrete examples of adoption. With occupancy, use, and post occupancy evaluation (POE) follow-up, design principles and knowledge are set in stone (pun intended).

In this type of "adoption", there are many examples: actual buildings included in Volume Two of the ADI report, as well as numerous dementia-specific new buildings and renovations of buildings in the US, Europe, the UK, Australia, and other countries.

The ADI WAR report's "Pioneers and innovators" chapter (Zeisel, 2020) describes actual projects designed and built to demonstrate and test principles and approaches in situ in the 1980s and 1990s. Space considerations preclude a description of the contribution of each building but they should be named as pioneers: ADaRDS, Tasmania; Aldersgate, South Australia; Anton Pieckhofje; Haarlem Netherlands; Le Cantou, France; Hasselknuten, Sweden; Hearthstone, Massachusetts, USA; Himawari, Ofenatu Japan; Moorside, Winchester, UK; Pepper Tree Lodge, Queanbeyan, Australia; and Woodside Place, Oakmont, PA, USA.

In the footsteps of these pioneers, Zeisel used this method to link dementia-specific knowledge to design, collaborating with architects designing, developing, and testing evidence-based buildings for elders and those living with dementia. These collaborations resulted in widely publicised award-winning buildings that illustrated the impact of knowledge adoption, including, among others:

Captain Clarence Eldridge House (Hyannis, MA) (Morton, 1981), Sterling Estates The Grande (Atlanta, GA), AHAVA Nursing Home conversion (Pittsburgh, PA), and Hearthstone Alzheimer Care neighbourhoods in Assisted Living Communities in the US – Hopkinton, Marlboro, Woburn (Zeisel, 2006, pp. 375–380), and Brockton, Massachusetts and Manhattan, Westchester, and Palisades, in New York state.

Adoption Case Study:

The following annotated plan of Sterling Estates' award-winning The Grande Memory Care community in Cobb County, Atlanta, illustrates how the built environment embodies and promotes adoption of evidence-based dementia design knowledge (Figure 13.2).

Stage four: adherence

Reaching adherence comes with time. New knowledge gains traction as it is used in publicised buildings that become recognised as best practice. New knowledge generates adherence when endorsed in handbooks, guidelines, and eventually in standards and regulation. This is not something that can be forced; rather requiring gradual establishment of trust in the new knowledge. Energetic and sustained efforts in establishing awareness, agreement, and adoption facilitates knowledge adherence.

Australia provides an excellent example of adherence to evidence-based dementia design knowledge through regulation and policy. For the past decade, government funded Dementia Training Australia (Dementia Training Australia) has employed the Principles as the basis for its education programs across Australia. In 2015 New South Wales Health adopted the Principles as key to improving healthcare environments for people living with dementia (Fleming & Bennett, 2014); in 2016 they were included in the Australasian Health Facility Guidelines for application to the design of mental health facilities for older people (AHIA, 2015) and referenced in the 2019 revision (Australasian Health Infrastructure Alliance, 2019); in 2018 they became the standard by which the Australian Aged Care Quality and Safety Commission

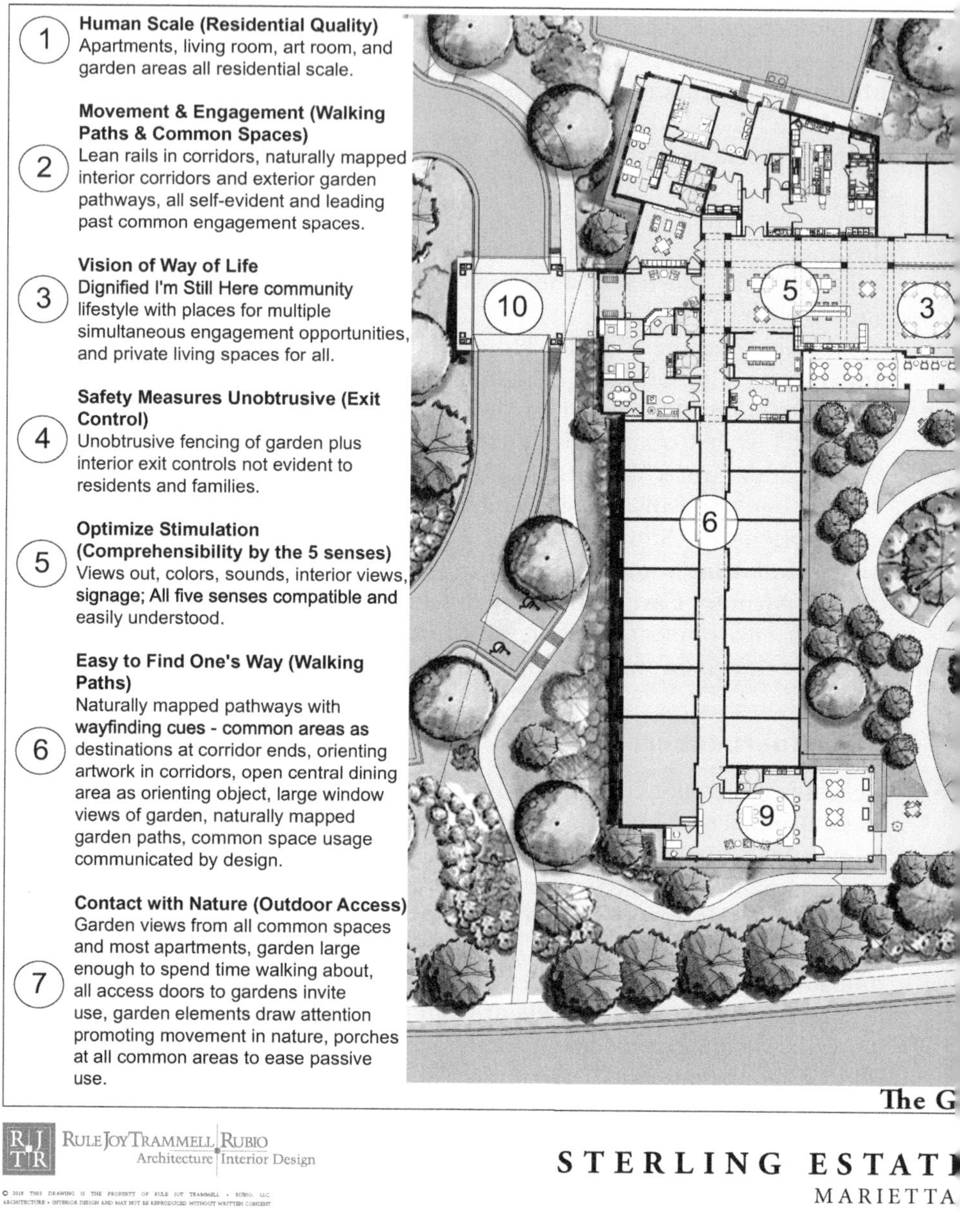

1 Human Scale (Residential Quality)
Apartments, living room, art room, and garden areas all residential scale.

2 Movement & Engagement (Walking Paths & Common Spaces)
Lean rails in corridors, naturally mapped interior corridors and exterior garden pathways, all self-evident and leading past common engagement spaces.

3 Vision of Way of Life
Dignified I'm Still Here community lifestyle with places for multiple simultaneous engagement opportunities, and private living spaces for all.

4 Safety Measures Unobtrusive (Exit Control)
Unobtrusive fencing of garden plus interior exit controls not evident to residents and families.

5 Optimize Stimulation (Comprehensibility by the 5 senses)
Views out, colors, sounds, interior views, signage; All five senses compatible and easily understood.

6 Easy to Find One's Way (Walking Paths)
Naturally mapped pathways with wayfinding cues - common areas as destinations at corridor ends, orienting artwork in corridors, open central dining area as orienting object, large window views of garden, naturally mapped garden paths, common space usage communicated by design.

7 Contact with Nature (Outdoor Access)
Garden views from all common spaces and most apartments, garden large enough to spend time walking about, all access doors to gardens invite use, garden elements draw attention promoting movement in nature, porches at all common areas to ease passive use.

The G

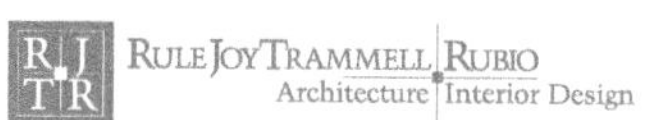

STERLING ESTAT
MARIETTA

Figure 13.2 © The Grande, Sterling Estates, Atlanta; Programming/Design Review: John Zeisel PhD & Marc A. Maxwell AIA; Architecture and Interior Design by Rule Joy Trammell + Rubio.

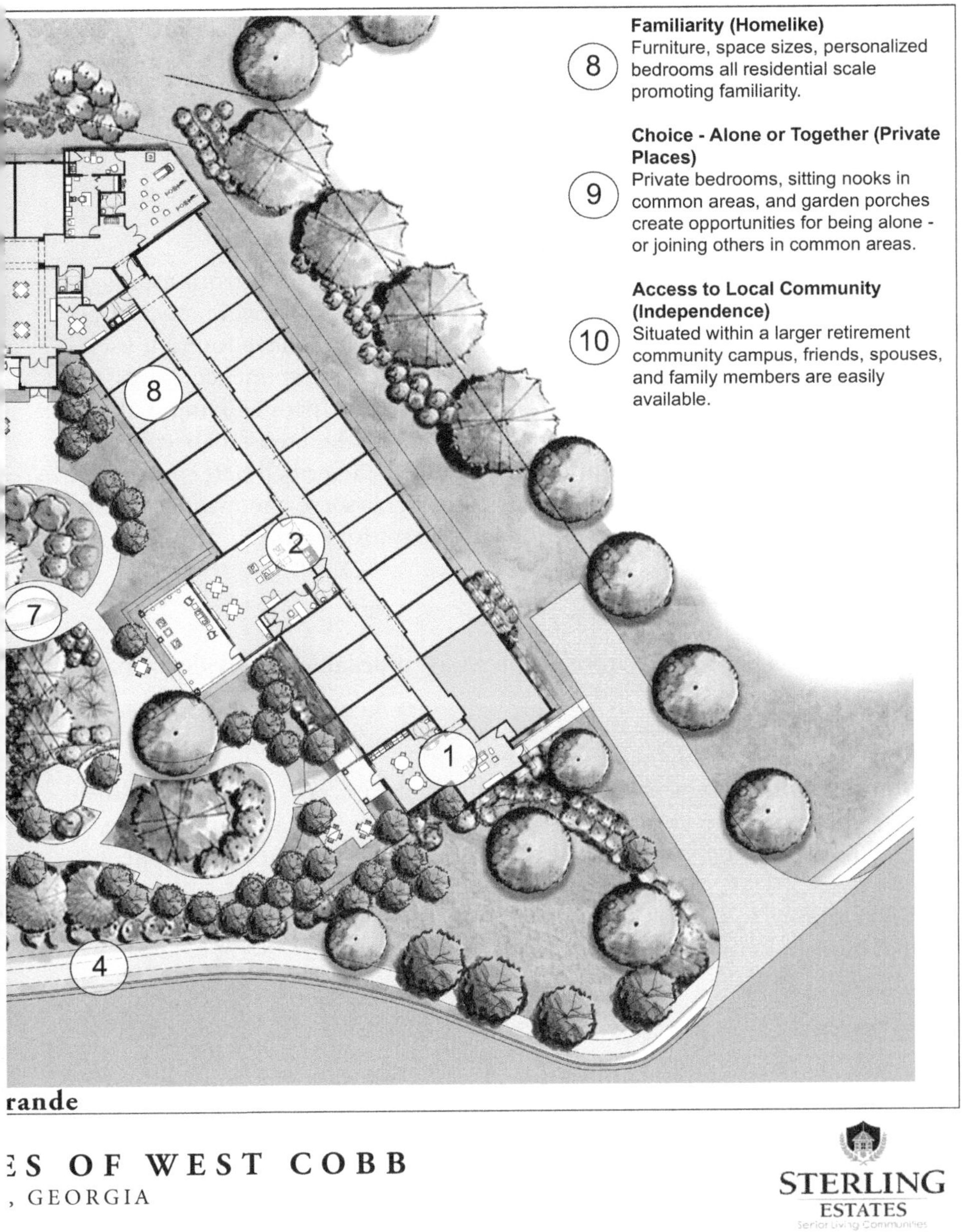

Familiarity (Homelike)
Furniture, space sizes, personalized bedrooms all residential scale promoting familiarity.

Choice - Alone or Together (Private Places)
Private bedrooms, sitting nooks in common areas, and garden porches create opportunities for being alone - or joining others in common areas.

Access to Local Community (Independence)
Situated within a larger retirement community campus, friends, spouses, and family members are easily available.

rande

S OF WEST COBB
, GEORGIA

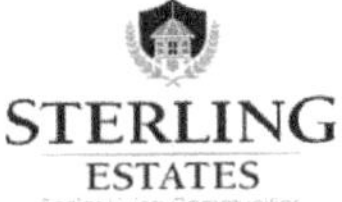
STERLING
ESTATES
Senior Living Communities

(ACQSC) judged design as evidenced by the resources provided for guidance (Aged Care Quality and safety Commission, 2018) and their influence has continued as the foundation for the new National Aged Care Design Principles and Guidelines (Seemann et al., 2023).

Present efforts to have dementia design principles included in National Dementia Plans represent another significant step towards adoption

Conclusion

While there is still a great deal more to achieve, the path from establishing consensual knowledge through the four stages of awareness, agreement, adoption, and adherence is ongoing. The authors have found it useful to look back on their activities through this lens. Experience raises the question – would the objectives of designing well for people living with dementia have been more effective had professionals taken as their collective approach to knowledge translation, the roadmap described here? And since the road does not end here, might this approach serve the evidence-based dementia design community as a productive path forward.

In-depth box

The authors describe their efforts to promote affordable and evidence-based design over a forty-year period by:

- Raising awareness of the available evidence.
- Working with design professionals and aged care providers to gain their agreement that the available knowledge called for a change in practice.
- Explaining through various means how the knowledge can be put into practice.
- Contributing to the development of guidelines and regulations to ensure that current knowledge is consistently applied.

References

Aged Care Quality and safety Commission. (2018). *Guidance and resources for providers to support the aged care quality standards. Organisation's service environment. Standard 5.* https://www.agedcarequality.gov.au/media/79920

AHIA. (2015). *Australasian health facility guidelines: Part B - Health facility briefing and planning, 0135- plder persons acute mental health unit.* Australasian Health Infrastructure Alliance. https://aushfg-prod-com-au.s3.amazonaws.com/HPU_B.0135_2_0.pdf

Australasian Health Infrastructure Alliance. (2019). *Australasian health facility guidelines, Part B - health facility briefing and planning, 135 – older peoples acute mental health inpatient unit.* https://healthfacilityguidelines.com.au/health-planning-units

Bennett, K., Fleming, R., & Zeisel, J. (2020). Design Principles and their use in this report. In R. Fleming, J. Zeisel, & K. Bennett (Eds.), *World Alzheimer Report 2020: Design Dignity Dementia, dementia-related design and the built environment* (Vol. 1, pp. 25–46). Alzheimer's Disease International.

Blythe, R., & Nazareth, I. (Eds.). (2017). *Dementia Studios*. RMIT.

Calkins, M. P. (1988.). *Design for dementia: Planning environments for the elderly and the confused*. National Health Publishing.

Charras, K., Eynard, C., & Viatour, G. (2016). Use of space and Human Rights: Planning dementia friendly settings. *Journal of Gerontological Social Work, 59*(3), 181–204.

Chaudhury, H., Cooke, H. A., Cowie, H., & Razaghi, L. (2018). The influence of the physical environment on residents with dementia in long-term care settings: A review of the empirical literature. *Gerontologist, 58*(5), e325–e337.

Cohen, U., & Weisman, G.D. (1991). *Holding on to home: Designing environments for people with dementia*. Johns Hopkins University Press.

Dementia Training Australia. *Environments Consultancy*. https://dta.com.au/services/#environments

Draper, B., Low, L.-F., Withall, A., Vickland, V., & Ward, T. (2009). Translating dementia research into practice. *International Psychogeriatrics, 21*(SupplementS1), S72–S80. https://doi.org/10.1017/S1041610209008709

Farrow, M., Doherty, K., McInerney, F., Klekociuk, S. Z., Bindoff, A., & Vickers, J. C. (2018). Improving knowledge and practice through massive open online dementia education: The understanding dementia and preventing dementia MOOCs. *Alzheimer's & Dementia, 14*(7), 233–233. https://doi.org/10.1016/j.jalz.2018.06.2368

Fleming, R. (2011). An environmental audit tool suitable for use in homelike facilities for people with dementia. *Australasian Journal on Ageing, 30*(3), 108–112. https://doi.org/10.1111/j.1741-6612.2010.00444.x

Fleming, R., & Bennett, K. (2014). *Key principles for improving healthcare environments for people with dementia*. Agency for Clinical Innovation, NSW Ministry of Health. http://www.aci.health.nsw.gov.au/__data/assets/pdf_file/0019/280270/ACI_Key_Principles_for_Improving_Healthcare_Environments_for_People_with_Dementia.PDF

Fleming, R., & Bennett, K. (2015). Assessing the quality of environmental design of nursing homes for people with dementia: Development of a new tool. *Australasian Journal on Ageing, 34*(3), 191–194. https://doi.org/10.1111/ajag.12233

Fleming, R., & Bennett, K. (2019). *Environmental design resources*. Dementia Training Australia. Retrieved August 25, 2021, from https://dta.com.au/resources/environmental-design-resources-introduction/

Fleming, R., & Bowles, J. (1987, November). Units for the confused and disturbed elderly: Development, Design, Programmimg and Evaluation. *Australian Journal on Ageing, 6*(4), 25–28.

Fleming, R., Forbes, I., & Bennett, K. (2003). *Adapting the ward for people with dementia*. NSW Department of Health.

Fleming, R., Goodenough, B., Low, L.-F., Chenoweth, L., & Brodaty, H. (2016). The relationship between the quality of the built environment and the quality of life of people with dementia in residential care. *Dementia (14713012), 15*(4), 663–680. https://doi.org/10.1177/1471301214532460

Fleming, R., & Purandare, N. (2010, November). Long-term care for people with dementia: Environmental design guidelines. *International Psychogeriatrics*, 22(7), 1084–1096. https://doi.org/10.1017/s1041610210000438

Fleming, R., Zeisel, J., & Bennett, K. (2020). *Design Dignity dementia: Dementia-related design and the built environment. Volume I* World Alzheimer Report 2020, Issue. https://www.alz.co.uk/u/WorldAlzheimerReport2020Vol1.pdf

Fleming, R., Zeisel, J., & Bennett, K. (2021). *The Dignity Manifesto of Design for people living with dementia*. Design Dignity Dementia Organisation. Retrieved August 25, 2021, from https://designdignitydementia.com/

Golembiewski, J. A. (2020). Dementia-related design in the national dementia plans. In R. Fleming, J. Zeisel, & K. Bennett (Eds.), *Design dignity dementia: Dementia-related design and the built environment.* (Vol. 1, pp. 106–111). Alzheimers Disease International. https://www.alzint.org/resource/world-alzheimer-report-2020/

Hatcher, D., Chang, E., Schmied, V., & Garrido, S. (2019, June 18). Exploring the perspectives of older people on the concept of home. *Journal of Aging Research*, *2019*, 2679680. https://doi.org/10.1155/2019/2679680

Lawton, M. P. (1990). Environmental approaches to research and treatment of Alzheimer's Disease. In E. Light & B. D. Lebowitz (Eds.), *Treatment and family stress: Directions for research*. National Institute of Mental Health, U.S. Department of Health and Human Services.

Marcello, F., Buckley, P., Sugiyama, T., & Wesselius, H. (2015, October 2–3). *Design for dementia: Exploring alternative places, spaces and practices of care.* 8th International Conference and Exhibition of the Association of Architecture Schools of Australasia, Christchurch, New Zealand. https://www.academia.edu/18967819/Design_for_Dementia_Exploring_Alternative_Places_Spaces_and_Practices_of_Care?email_work_card=view-paper

Marshall, M. (2001). Environment: How it helps to see dementia as a disability. In S. Benson (Ed.), *Care homes and dementia*. The Journal of Dementia Care.

Morton, D. (1981, August). Captain clarence eldridge house, Hyannis, Ma.--congregate living. *Prog Arch*, *62*(8), 64–68.

Pathman, D. E., Konrad, T. R., Freed, G. L., Freeman, V. A., & Koch, G. G. (1996, September). The awareness-to-adherence model of the steps to clinical guideline compliance. The case of pediatric vaccine recommendations. *Medical Care*, *34*(9), 873–889.

Quirke, M., Ostwald, M., Fleming, R., Taylor, M., & Williams, A. (2023). A design assessment tool for layout planning in residential care for dementia. *Architectural Science Review*, *66*(2), 122–132. https://doi.org/10.1080/00038628.2021.1984869

Seemann, N., Fuggle, L., Week, D., A., W., Morris, D., Loggie, C., Thompson, C., Fildes, D., Grootemaat, P., Lambourne, S., Goodenough, B., & Gordon, R. (2023). *Final report on the development of the national aged care design principles and guidelines*.

United Nations. (2019). *World population ageing 2019: Highlights*. www.un.org/en/development/desa/population/publications/pdf/ageing/WorldPopulationAgeing2019-Highlights.pdf

Zeisel, J. (1984). *Inquiry by design: Tools for environment-behavior research*. Cambridge University Press. https://search.library.wisc.edu/catalog/999553259602121

Zeisel, J. (2006). *Inquiry by design: Environment/behavior/neuroscience in architecture, interiors, landscape, and planning.* W W Norton & Co.

Zeisel, J. (2010). *I'm Still Here: A breakthrough approach to understanding someone living with Alzheimer's.* Piatkus.

Zeisel, J. (2020). Dementia care design: Groundbreakers and lessons learned. In R. Fleming, J. Zeisel, & K. Bennett (Eds.), *World Alzheimer Report 2020: Design dignity dementia, dementia-related design and the built environment* (Vol. 1). Alzheimer's Disease International.

Zeisel, J., Hyde, J., & Levkoff, S. (1994, March/April, 4). Best practices: An Environment Behavior (EB) model for Alzheimer special care units. *American Journal of Alzheimer's Care and Related Disorders and Research*, 21.

Zeisel, J., Reisberg, B., Whitehouse, P., Woods, R., & Verheul, A. (2016). Ecopsychosocial interventions in cognitive decline and dementia: A new terminology and a new paradigm. *American Journal of Alzheimer's Disease and Other Dementias*, 31(6), 502–507.

14

Sociotherapeutic living environments in long-term care organisations

*Debby Gerritsen, Hanneke Noordam,
Hanneke Nijsten and Hanneke Donkers*

Introduction (research area and problem statement)

In the distant past, care organisations mainly offered undifferentiated care based on a medical model of care applying the diagnosis as a description of cause and effect, independent of the social environment (Janzing & Kerstens, 2012). Nowadays, residents of a long-term care organisation in the Netherlands, including people with dementia, receive multidisciplinary care, nursing, treatment and support (Koopmans et al., 2022). They often have highly complex care and support needs. Ideally, optimal quality of life for the resident is the starting point for good, demand-driven care and support that meets the wishes and needs of people with dementia. This care takes shape in the interaction between resident, informal carer and healthcare professional, at the location where the resident lives. Demand-driven care, support, housing and well-being are therefore closely interrelated (Chaudhury et al., 2018; de Boer et al., 2018).

In several care organisations in the Netherlands, demand-driven care is operationalised by working with sociotherapeutic living environments (STLs). An STL is a living environment providing a context adapted to the residents' *current* needs, abilities, behaviours and cognitive level. These current needs, abilities and behaviour often differ from these prior to diagnosis. The resident can enter relationships with fellow residents, informal carers, volunteers and care professionals in a safe and appropriate environment. Through this, opportunities arise for creating an environment in which the resident can achieve optimal functioning despite ones physical, cognitive and social problems that arise in many areas of life. In STLs, residents are grouped in one of several environments, based on their (care) needs and wishes regarding social environment (individual or group orientated), activity and rest, amount of structure and directiveness, social interaction, involvement in society, and safety. There are four main STLs which vary in physical layout, level of environmental stimuli, nature and type of activities, and personal approach (Table 14.1). Based on their existing or endeavoured competences, preferences and skills nursing staff members are also selected for one of the environments (van Tiel et al., 2012).

DOI: 10.4324/9781003416241-20

Table 14.1 Central aspects of the four living environments

Balance group	Physical layout	Individual or small group; lay-out is a combination of communal space and more private corners.
	Stimuli/ activities	Balancing daily routine rest - activity, balancing social interaction group - individual time in own room.
	Personal approach	Providing structure and guidance with empathic-directive approach. Supporting tasks of daily living and domestic activities.
Atmosphere group	Physical layout	Small group; lay-out is warm, comforting and individually oriented.
	Stimuli/ activities	Rest, tranquil atmosphere.
	Personal approach	Providing physical and psychological safety for individual and group, by means of an empathic, warm, and sheltering approach, taking over tasks of daily living and domestic activities.
Socio group	Physical layout	Lay-out is open, inviting and facilitates group process (big tables).
	Stimuli/ activities	Stimulating environment; participating in domestic activities, e.g., cooking, taking care of plants.
	Personal approach	Providing stimulation for social engagement and engaging approach for social and domestic activities.
Beacon group	Physical layout	Individual; clear lay-out; individually orientated by creating 1-person seats. Calm interior.
	Stimuli/ activities	Focus on reducing stimuli, mostly individual activities or domestic chores.
	Personal approach	Providing an empathic directive approach; a clear structure, routines and regularity, providing directives and boundaries. Aimed at prevention of agitation and challenging behaviour.

STLs has its origins in psychiatry (Hirsch, 2001; Janzing & Kerstens, 2012; Lawton, 1986). In the Netherlands, attention to the possibilities of sociotherapy in the care for people with dementia was first paid in 1981 (Luijten, 1981). Yet, a first specific application of sociotherapeutic environments within dementia care was only published in 2007 by the Steering Group for people with Young Onset Dementia (Stuurgroep jong dementerenden, 2007). In 2012, the long-term care organisation Archipel published a guide to sociotherapeutic living environments that focused on the residents with Gerontopsychiatric conditions, Korsakov's disease and people with Young Onset Dementia (van Tiel et al., 2012). At least five other long-term care organisations have since then started the implementation of STLs.

Care organisations in the Netherlands that work with sociotherapeutic environments do so from a practice-based perspective, as empirical evaluations are lacking. In this chapter, we provide insight into the principles of sociotherapeutic environments based on a literature review of practice documentation on STLs and of scientific papers. We integrate the findings into a theoretical framework for the application of sociotherapeutic environments in the care of people with dementia. Furthermore, we describe action research that we conducted to evaluate and possibly improve the current work processes, elements and implementation of STLs (Donkers, in preparation).

State of the art review (what do we know)

Practice documentation

In 2017, we performed a review of practice and scientific documentation (Noordam, 2019). As a first step, the six care organisations known to the authors of having STLs were approached via email and requested to share their practical documents on STLs. Four of these shared practice documents, e.g., developed manuals and care programs. We studied the provided practice documentation for elements of STLs and identified the following:

Content principles: there is a lot of overlap between the organisations' principles, as they are all based on the 2007 Steering Group document (Stuurgroep jong dementerenden, 2007) or Archipel's guide (van Tiel et al., 2012). In their vision on care, all organisations mention resident centeredness and/ or demand-driven care: the wishes and needs of people with dementia are the central starting point. A group of residents is composed based on corresponding needs and care requirements within four life domains: living environment, participation; mental and physical well-being. The organisations also broadly distinguish the same types of STLs as identified in Archipel's guide; socio group, atmosphere group, beacon group and balance group (see Table 14.1). Depending on the residents present, there are sometimes additional STLs or the orientation of the STLs may differ. For instance, one organisation uses three instead of four STLs named mood group ('nurturing' environment), beacon group ('empowering' environment) and balance group ('structuring' environment).

Differentiating residents: most organisations differentiate first by diagnosis and second by care needs. Three organisations use a placement list with criteria, concerning needs for social interaction, level of support needed, stimuli and structure. Others make a choice for an STL based on information acquired at registration and/or a meeting with the new resident and their informal carer. Several organisations perform a home visit prior to admitment in nursing home based on which placement recommendation follows.

Nursing staff selection: all organisations differentiate nursing staff according to their competencies for the various STLs. At one of the long-term care organisations, the different types of STLs were simulated when the concept was implemented so that employees could experience which environment they would feel most comfortable with.

Open or more closed STLs: Four of the six organisations implemented a more "open" model, so that residents could move between STLs during the day depending on their needs and interests. At one organisation, the resident's bedroom is deliberately not linked to a specific living environment, in order to achieve the most flexible concept possible and which allows a new resident to be placed immediately when a bedroom becomes available. At the other three organisations, however, the bedroom is located within the STL.

Embedding of STLs: five of the six organisations have defined implementation and sustainment strategies, including an STL expert team, appointing a subject specialist for each team, a regular STL meeting, developing information leaflets, involving family members, involvement of a quality officer, coaching on the job, regular evaluations or audits on working with STLs and setting up working group(s) to implement improvements.

Published studies

Furthermore, to gain insight into the principles of STLs, a literature search was carried out in PubMed in November 2018 (Noordam, 2019). The following search terms were used: dementia, Alzheimer's, sociotherapy, Socioenvironmental Therapy, Nurse-Patient relations, Residential Facilities, Health Services for the Aged, long-term care organisation. This resulted in 191 publications. Titles and abstracts of these publications were screened by two authors and were selected if they related to sociotherapy or environmental therapy; the therapeutic influence of the living environment in an inpatient setting on residents (including people with dementia); needs of residents (including people with dementia) in relation to the living environment; possible contribution of the living environment to treatment and quality of life. Using the reference lists of the selected articles, a further search was conducted using the snowball method.

The literature on sociotherapy we found (Noordam, 2019) specifically appears to consist mainly of descriptive reports on specific programs or general articles on its principles and benefits (Probst, 2016). Empirical studies were scarce and of limited quality. The few studies on sociotherapy for people with dementia indicated positive results (Espinosa et al., 2015; Grasel et al., 2003; Hirsch, 2001), but the authors recommend larger-scale research (Grasel et al., 2003).

The following needs emerged in the literature on living environments for residents with dementia: need for structure (including structuring of stimuli), safety, autonomy, social contact, meaningful activity and family involvement (Calkins, 2018; Stuurgroep jong dementerenden, 2007; Stuurgroep jonge mensen met dementie, 2004; Helden & Bakker, 2017; Luijten, 1981; Taft et al., 1993). These needs can be translated into requirements or "therapeutic goals" for the social, physical and organisational living environment. For example, supporting privacy and security, recognizability, facilitating social contact, mobility, regulating stimulation (Calkins, 2018; Cohen, 1991).

Identified elements of the *physical environment* are design, atmosphere, functionality, orientation, balance between safety and autonomy and structuring/mediating environmental stimuli (Calkins, 2018; Helden & Bakker, 2017; Morgan & Stewart, 1999; Taft et al., 1993). Elements of the *social environment* that were identified are: structure, daily routine, activities, communication, autonomy, social relationships with fellow residents, family and staff, validating feelings and carer attitudes (Helden & Bakker, 2017; Morgan & Stewart, 1997). Elements of the *organisational environment*: number and disciplines of staff members and resources (e.g., form of housing, therapy rooms) (Claassen, 2014; Janzing & Kerstens, 2012). Furthermore, the interaction between the resident and these elements of the STL is consciously and therapeutically employed. Prerequisites here are: a unified approach from the team and good communication between team members, family and residents.

By tailoring and applying these elements, the needs and goals of the resident can be fulfilled. The interaction between the resident and their environment is used consciously and therapeutically with the ultimate goal to optimise Quality of Life (Calkins, 2018; Cohen, 1991; Morgan & Stewart, 1997, 1999; Taft et al., 1993).

We integrated these insights from the literature on living environments for residents with dementia with the conceptual models of Cohen and Weisman (Cohen, 1991) and Morgan and Stewart (Morgan & Stewart, 1997), into a conceptual model of STLs in the care of people with dementia (see Figure 14.1).

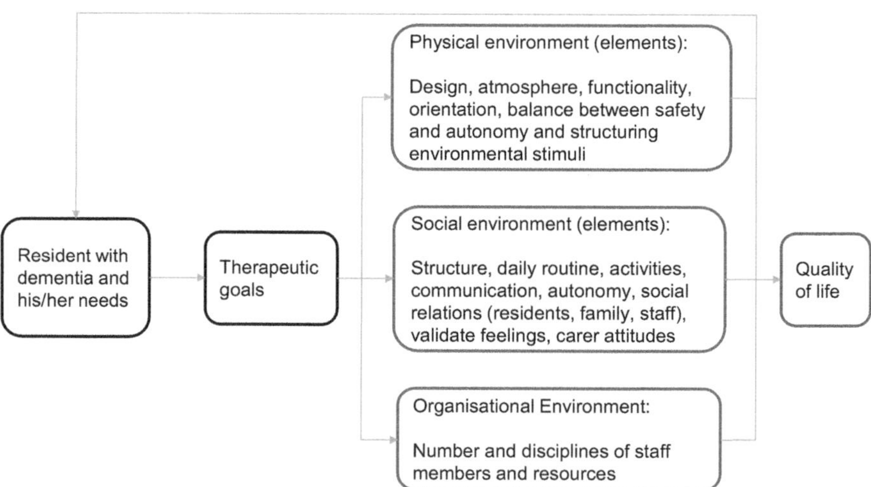

Figure 14.1 Conceptual model of sociotherapeutic living environments in the care of people with dementia

Living environments for residents with dementia and person-centred care

In STLs, the resident's needs are the starting point for developing an appropriate therapeutic living environment, with the goal of positively influencing quality of life. Having the resident's needs as a starting point also holds for person-centred care and quality of life approaches (Gerritsen, 2023; Kitwood, 1997). According to Kitwood's person-centred care approach, one contributes to the quality of life of people with dementia by matching care to the individual's abilities, needs, desires and habits. Kitwood identifies five basic psychological needs of people with dementia: attachment, comfort, identity and self-esteem, being involved/ having something to do and belonging (Kitwood, 1997; Kitwood & Bredin, 1992). According to Kitwood, these needs are universal but are greater in people with dementia, as people with dementia are more vulnerable and less able to act on these needs themselves (Mitchell & Agnelli, 2015). The quality of nursing staff and the care environment therefore determine whether and to what extent the psychological needs of people with dementia are met, and as such can contribute to maintaining or increasing quality of life (Mitchell & Agnelli, 2015). The empirical literature on (unmet) needs of people with dementia shows that meeting needs of residents can contribute to quality of life, although several studies suggest that the focus in a long-term care organisation still tends to be on the physical health needs of people with dementia and that needs for meaningfulness and social well-being are more often left unmet (Cadieux et al., 2013; Hancock et al., 2006; Shiells et al., 2020). Cohen-Mansfield's review (Cohen-Mansfield et al., 2015) supports these findings and specifically describes a high prevalence of unmet needs when it comes to loneliness, need for social contact, boredom, need for meaningful activities and various types of discomfort. Unmet needs, in turn, are associated with challenging behaviours and can lower quality of life (Hancock et al., 2006). Although STLs seem to respond to relevant needs in terms of quality of life, the question remains to what extent there is room for the psychological need 'attachment' (Kitwood, 1997) in the composition of the STL groups, since the focus in STLs seems to mainly be on care-related problems and needs.

Action research

To evaluate and possibly improve the current work processes, elements, and implementation of STLs an action research project was designed according to the action research cycle PLAN-ACT-OBSERVE-REFLECT (Cardiff & van Lieshout, 2017). Action research is an approach to research that aims both to improve daily practice and to develop knowledge about that improvement applying a cyclical approach in which stakeholders participate (Cardiff & van Lieshout, 2017). In our study, 34 residents and informal carers – representing their loved ones who lived with dementia – and 34 care professionals from 11 STLs from two different care organisations participated in the study. Several of them were actively involved in the design of the study and at every stage of its execution. The project ran two cycles (Donkers, in preparation).

The observation and reflection phases of cycle one showed no additional needs that should be addressed, but respondents mentioned it being important to map the resident's life history, preferences and habits in addition to identifying needs and care preferences as well as addressing the resident's social well-being. Furthermore, it appeared that both informal carers and staff were predominantly satisfied with the current situation of living in and working with STLs and prefer this to not living or working in STLs. Continuous education of care professionals and an increase of family involvement were considered necessary. People also mentioned the importance of further STL-specific concretization of the physical and social environment, such as furnishings and a further tailoring of the provided activities. As for the organisational environment, optimising the process of placement required attention, as well as ensuring continuity, for example of staffing and of the personal approach by staff.

The observation and reflection phases of cycle 2, carried out after the plan and action phases in which the areas for improvement on each location were prioritized and implemented as discussed in the evaluation meetings, showed that there was increased awareness among staff of their working in STLs and that various change processes had been initiated: establishment of a working group on furnishing, exploration of cooperating with designers, optimisation of activities, optimisation of continuity of staff, optimisation of the process of resident placement. Furthermore, concrete tools had been developed: an optimised placement form and information materials for relatives, and an e-learning module (Donkers, in preparation).

General considerations

The (care) needs of residents are the starting point in working with STLs. These needs can be translated into therapeutic goals for the social and physical environment. By specifically deploying elements of the social and physical environment, these therapeutic goals can be addressed with the goal of optimising quality of life. The elements of the organisational environment facilitate implementation and sustainment of the STLs. The elements of the social, physical and organisational environment inventoried in the literature are broadly consistent with the elements mentioned by participants in our action research. STLs were further found to be consistent with a person-centred care approach. Comparison with the literature on person-centred care shows that STLs seem to respond to relevant needs in terms of quality of life (Kitwood, 1997; Probst, 2016), although the need 'attachment' requires additional attention because the focus in the composition of the STL groups seems to mainly be on problems and care-related needs. Co-residents are an important source of attachment, but in the current set-up it is quite possible, for example, that two residents who are similar in their need for structure and type of treatment, do not get along at all and find it difficult to live together in an STL. As such, differentiation on care needs may imply that there is less room for a personal match. Furthermore, the importance emerged of giving residents choices within or between the STL regarding levels of social interaction, stimulation and activities. This deserves further research as preferences of a resident may be at odds with what others involved regard as contributing to the quality of life of the resident and/or his fellow residents.

Recommendations

Practice

STLs appear to be a promising methodology for long-term care for people with dementia. Further concretization of residents' needs per STL and a unified way to record them is, however, recommended. Systematic and regular mapping of residents' needs makes explicit what care should be focused on and can contribute significantly to their quality of life. Furthermore, the needs of a resident may change, and it is important that the STL concept offers sufficient flexibility for this, in both the physical environment (e.g., offering choice in types of environments), the social environment (e.g., type of activities, dynamics) and the organisational environment (e.g., deployment of staff).

A next recommendation is to take more account of a personal match between residents when placing them. However, this placement process in STLs is already complex and can be at odds with the logistics of care organisations; the far-reaching differentiation can lead to waiting lists for the right STL, empty places in case of mismatches of STL and residents and thus increase the likelihood of financial strain. Our recommendation further complicates this. However, this study did find existing variations of STLs that could reduce the impact on operations, such as more open STLs where residents' bedrooms are not linked to the STL and establishing a first entry unit where one can get to know a new resident without great time pressure, before selecting a type of STL.

Regarding the physical environment, further elaboration proved necessary, which may address light, sound, interior design as well as garden- and landscaping. A way to do this is taken up in our current study (Donkers et al., in preparation) and involves specialized designers (e.g., interior designer / architect, sound designer, garden and landscape architect) and together work out and apply possibilities for the physical environment of the various types of STLs.

Future research

Future research directions include the further specification and evaluation of the elements, working mechanisms and implementation strategies of STLS in daily practice. Next to specifically addressing the implications of care needs for the design of the physical environment, increasing attention is needed for participation of family carers, continuous education of care professionals and further specification of daily activities per living environment. Furthermore, the contribution of STLs to the wellbeing of residents, family and professionals needs investigation. More clarity on the effects of differentiation on diagnosis, care demand and/or identity on the (social) well-being of long-term care organisation residents is also of great value.

Further empirical research can provide insight into the effects of STLs on the quality of care provided and the quality of life of residents. Furthermore, effects of working in STLs on staff members need investigation. Having satisfied employees is extremely relevant to a care organisation, especially in today's tight labour market with high turnover and vacancies. Working in STLs, in which placement is based on staff's competencies and preferences, could contribute to this.

In-depth box

- STLS are demand driven and residents are grouped in one of several environments, based on their current (care) needs and wishes regarding social and physical environment. STLs address resident needs adequately and provide the resident with a safe and appropriate environment according to (informal) carers.
- Care professionals are selected for one of the environments based on their competences, preferences and skills. (Informal) carers report more continuity in provided care and a more stable environment.
- By involving (informal) carers and when possible, persons with dementia in our action research on STLS, we included a specific perspective that is very relevant for improving quality of life.

References

Cadieux, M. A., Garcia, L. J., & Patrick, J. (2013). Needs of people with dementia in long-term care: A systematic review. *American Journal of Alzheimers Disease and Other Dementias, 28*(8), 723–733. https://doi.org/10.1177/1533317513500840

Calkins, M. P. (2018). From research to application: Supportive and therapeutic environments for people living with dementia. *Gerontologist, 58*, S114–S128. https://doi.org/10.1093/geront/gnx146

Cardiff, J. &, van Lieshout, F. (2017). *Actieonderzoek: principes voor verandering in zorg en welzijn* (1st ed.). Koninklijke Van Gorkum, Assen.

Chaudhury, H., Cooke, H. A., Cowie, H., & Razaghi, L. (2018). The influence of the physical environment on residents with dementia in long-term care settings:

A review of the empirical literature. *Gerontologist, 58*(5), e325–e337. https://doi. org/10.1093/geront/gnw259

Claassen, A. e. J. C. (2014). Het effect van samenhangend behandelen: Introductie van een model voor multidisciplinair werken in de GGz *Groepen, 9*(4), 25–40.

Cohen, W. (1991). *Holding on to home. Designing environments for people with dementia.* Johns Hopkins University Press.

Cohen-Mansfield, J., Dakheel-Ali, M., Marx, M. S., Thein, K., & Regier, N. G. (2015). Which unmet needs contribute to behavior problems in persons with advanced dementia? *Psychiatry Research, 228*(1), 59–64. https://doi.org/10.1016/j. psychres.2015.03.043

de Boer, B., Beerens, H. C., Katterbach, M. A., Viduka, M., Willemse, B. M., & Verbeek, H. (2018). The physical environment of nursing homes for people with dementia: Traditional nursing homes, small-scale living facilities, and green care farms. *Healthcare (Basel), 6*(4). https://doi.org/10.3390/healthcare6040137

Donkers, H., Noordam, H., Matser, A., & Gerritsen, D. (in preparation). Development and evaluation of an intervention to enhance the physical environment of nursing homes: A feasibility study.

Donkers, H., Leontjevas, R., Nijsten, H., Koopmans, R., & Gerritsen, D. (in preparation). How to align the physical environment to the needs of residents with dementia in long-term care setting: Action research on sociotherapeutic environments.

Espinosa, L., Harris, B., Frank, J., Armstrong-Muth, J., Brous, E., Moran, J., & Giorgi-Cipriano, J. (2015). Milieu improvement in psychiatry using evidence-based practices: The long and winding road of culture change. *Archives of Psychiatric Nursing, 29*(4), 202–207. https://doi.org/10.1016/j.apnu.2014.08.004

Gerritsen, D. L. (2023). Well-being in long-term care: An ode to vulnerability. *Aging Ment Health, 27*(2), 230–235. https://doi.org/10.1080/13607863.2021.2008869

Grasel, E., Wiltfang, J., & Kornhuber, J. (2003). Non-drug therapies for dementia: An overview of the current situation with regard to proof of effectiveness. *Dementia and Geriatric Cognitive Disorders, 15*(3), 115–125. https://doi.org/10.1159/000068477

Hancock, G. A., Woods, B., Challis, D., & Orrell, M. (2006). The needs of older people with dementia in residential care. *International Journal of Geriatric Psychiatry, 21*(1), 43–49. https://doi.org/10.1002/gps.1421

Helden, M. v., & Bakker, T. (2017). Woon- en leefomgeving vanuit sociotherapeutisch perspectief. In *Klinisch redeneren bij ouderen: functiebehoud in levensloopperspectief.* Bohn Stafleu van Loghum.

Hirsch, R. D. (2001). Socio- and psychotherapy in patients with Alzheimer disease. *Zeitschrift für Gerontologie und Geriatrie, 34*(2), 92–100 (Sozio- und Psychotherapie bei Alzheimerkranken). https://www.ncbi.nlm.nih.gov/pubmed/11393010

Janzing, C., & Kerstens, J. (2012). *Werken in een therapeutisch milieu. Naar samenhangend behandelen in de GGz.* Bohn-Stafleu van Loghum.

Kitwood, T., & Bredin, K. (1992). Towards a theory of dementia care: Personhood and well-being. *Ageing & Society, 12*, 269–287.

Kitwood, T. M. (1997). *Dementia reconsidered: The person comes first.* Open University Press.

Koopmans, R., Leerink, B., & Festen, D. A. M. (2022). Dutch long-term care in transition: A guide for other countries. *Journal of the American Medical Directors Association, 23*(2), 204–206. https://doi.org/10.1016/j.jamda.2021.09.013

Lawton, M. P. (1986). *Environment and aging.* Center for the Study of Aging.

Luijten, J. J. (1981). Sociotherapie in een psychogeriatrisch verpleeghuis: ijdele hoop of hopeloze ijdelheid? *Tijdschrift voor psychiatrie 23*(5), 290–299.

Mitchell, G., & Agnelli, J. (2015). Person-centred care for people with dementia: Kitwood reconsidered. *Nurs Stand, 30*(7), 46–50. https://doi.org/10.7748/ns.30.7.46.s47

Morgan, D. G., & Stewart, N. J. (1997). The importance of the social environment in dementia care. *Western Journal of Nursing Research, 19*(6), 740–761. https://doi.org/10.1177/019394599701900604

Morgan, D. G., & Stewart, N. J. (1999). The physical environment of special care units: Needs of residents with dementia from the perspective of staff and family caregivers. *Qualitative Health Research, 9*(1), 105–118. https://doi.org/10.1177/104973299129121721

Noordam, H & Gerritsen, G. (2019). *De LIVE-studie: Een actieonderzoek naar sociotherapeutische leefmilieus in verpleeghuizen.* UKON.

Probst, B. (2016). Person-centered sociotherapy. In J. E. Mezzich, M. Botbol, G. N. Christodoulou, C. R. Cloninger, & I. M. Salloum (Eds.), *Person centered psychiatry* (pp. 263–275). Springer International Publishing. https://doi.org/10.1007/978-3-319-39724-5_20

Shiells, K., Pivodic, L., Holmerova, I., & Van den Block, L. (2020). Self-reported needs and experiences of people with dementia living in nursing homes: A scoping review. *Aging and Mental Health, 24*(10), 1553–1568. https://doi.org/10.1080/13607863.2019.1625303

Stuurgroep jong dementerenden. (2007). *Sociotherapeutische leefmilieus voor jong dementerenden.* Buro Salari.

Stuurgroep jonge mensen met dementie. (2004). *Landelijk Zorgprogramma Jong Dementerenden.* Buro Salari.

Taft, L. B., Delaney, K., Seman, D., & Stansell, J. (1993). Dementia care creating a therapeutic milieu. *Journal of Gerontological Nursing, 19*(10), 30–39. https://www.ncbi.nlm.nih.gov/pubmed/8409249

van Tiel, v. S., van Brug, R., & Jongeneelen, N. (2012). *Functieprogramma Sociotherapeutische Leefmilieus.* Archipel.

15

Dementia-friendly design

Towards minimizing spatial disorientation in residential care homes

Elena Carbone, Laura Miola, Erika Borella and Francesca Pazzaglia

Wayfinding: the cognitive and environmental psychology perspective

Wayfinding, that is, the process of determining and navigating a route from origin to destination (Golledge et al., 1987), represents a crucial ability in everyday life to undertake a great number of activities, both in outdoor and indoor environments.

Theoretical models grounded within the cognitive and environmental psychology highlight how finding the way in buildings is a complex, multicomponent ability derived from the interplay between different factors (Jamshidi et al., 2020). According to Carpman and Grant (2002), for example, individual factors (e.g., cognitive processes and individual differences like age and gender) and building design and elements (e.g., spatial layout, indoor signage, you-are-here maps, etc.) interact to make an environment easy to navigate and support indoor wayfinding behaviours. Carlson et al. (2010) also posited that indoor wayfinding complexity is determined by environmental variables (a building's features), people's spatial representations or cognitive maps (an internal representation, or mental image, of the environment; Tolman, 1948), and personal factors (an individual's spatial abilities and strategies).

The interplay between such elements, in terms of building–cognitive map correspondence, building–individual's strategies compatibility, and cognitive map–individual's spatial abilities and strategies completeness, explains navigation issues posed by a given building.

Overall, wayfinding is susceptible to broad individual differences that can be accounted for by factors intrinsic to individuals, such as their sensory-motor and cognitive abilities (e.g., memory and spatial abilities, problem-solving) and attitudes (e.g., sense of direction, spatial self-efficacy, pleasure in exploring, environment representation mode, and wayfinding strategies). Environmental attributes also play a key role in the wayfinding process. Wayfinding problems have the potential to impact individuals' physiological and psychological states. For instance, not being able to find a destination has been found

DOI: 10.4324/9781003416241-21

to be associated with higher blood pressure, increased physical aggression, and fatigue in healthcare settings (Carpman & Grant, 2002). It particularly applies to individuals with sensory impairments, limited physical mobility, and cognitive impairment, which includes people with dementia (PwD).

Wayfinding, aging, and dementia: the case of residential care homes

Wayfinding abilities are particularly sensitive to aging (e.g., Klencklen et al., 2012; Lester et al., 2017). Older adults encounter difficulties to orient themselves and learn routes in new environments (e.g., Carbone et al., 2021b; Meneghetti et al., 2016; see van der Ham et al., 2020). Even after learning a novel environment, older adults are less efficient than their younger counterparts in planning new routes through it by using acquired spatial information (e.g., Harris & Wolbers, 2014). Such decline is even more marked in individuals with mild cognitive impairment (MCI) or dementia (Mitolo et al., 2013). Spatial disorientation indeed is one of the earliest markers of neurocognitive disorders (Salimi et al., 2018). Several findings even suggests that adults at a higher genetic risk of developing dementia, in particular Alzheimer's disease, show signs of navigation deficits decades before clinical manifestations (Coughlan et al., 2019; Kunz et al., 2015).

Wayfinding difficulties may become particularly problematic in the case of a relocation from one's own habitual environment to unfamiliar surroundings, such as a residential care home (Wiener & Pazzaglia, 2021). Relocation represents a significant life event for PwD, encompassing a complex process of adaptation to a new environment (Castle, 2001). Apart from acclimating to new structured, routinized, and communal living conditions, PwD also have to deal with a disrupted sense of continuity, self-identity, sense of attachment, and familiarity, as well as a lack of control and autonomy over the relocation (Brownie et al., 2014). Such a transition is known to elicit negative emotional states (confusion, anxiety, and depression), as well as a worsening of symptoms and adverse health effects (Ryman et al., 2019). Maladjustment to the new living location might impact PwD's quality of life and wellbeing (Böckerman et al., 2012).

Such cognitive, physical, and emotional vulnerabilities lead PwD to become increasingly dependent on their environment, as envisaged by the environmental docility hypothesis (Lawton, 1977). From a cognitive and environmental psychology perspective, cognitive interventions based on route learning have been offered as a promising approach to sustain navigation and some related skills (e.g., spatial memory) in residential care home residents (Mitolo et al., 2017). Psychosocial interventions based on cognitive stimulation also represent to date evidence-based instruments to support residual cognitive resources as well as quality of life in PwD living in long-term care facilities (Carbone et al., 2021a). Besides these intervention approaches, the key role of the physical environment for the care of PwD living in residential care homes is increasingly acknowledged. Well-designed, supportive physical environments have indeed shown to reduce their behavioural and psychological symptoms (e.g., wandering, agitation, anxiety, aggression), support remaining abilities, autonomy, and engagement in meaningful stimulating and social activities, and enhance wellbeing (see Chaudhury et al., 2018). As such, long-term facilities designed also to support spatial orientation and wayfinding among PwD would facilitate the transition and contribute to their autonomy and wellbeing in the new accommodation.

Design factors towards minimising spatial disorientation among people with dementia living in residential care homes

Among the characteristics of a building capable of supporting individuals' wayfinding abilities is navigability, such as the extent to which a destination can be reached with reasonable effort and time (Carpman & Grant, 2002), that concurs in determining the environmental quality of a built environment. There are certain features of the building and of its interior design capable of making it easy to navigate, in particular its layout complexity, the presence of signage, and differentiation of visual, spatial, or interior design features (Devlin, 2014).

Given the importance of wayfinding abilities for supporting PwD's autonomy and wellbeing, how the environmental quality of a building, in terms of navigability and its factors, minimize their spatial disorientation and wayfinding issues in residential care homes has received increasing attention (Chaudhury et al., 2018; Wiener & Pazzaglia, 2021). Evidence of strategies that could be applied to support wayfinding behaviours among older residents with dementia has been reported in commentaries or literature reviews, quantitative studies using questionnaires, and some qualitative data studies (e.g., thematic analysis; O'Malley et al., 2018; Tao et al., 2018; Wiener & Pazzaglia, 2021).

Regarding the architecture of residential care homes, the complexity of layout in terms of size or number of floors has been shown to affect how legible the environment is (Baskaya et al., 2004). For example, a study using space syntax techniques for the analysis of spatial configurations in a residential care home showed that increasing complexity in the floor plan (e.g., increasing numbers of turns) was negatively associated with wayfinding and satisfaction of older residents (Tao et al., 2018). Furthermore, long corridors, continuous paths, and repetitive architectural features seem to not help orientation within residential care homes (Chaudhury et al., 2018; Marquardt, 2011). These results are consistent with a study that interviewed older adults who reported that walking long distances from the residential room to the common areas, with a sequence of doors all looking the same and without progressive numbering of the rooms, can make it more challenging for older adults to find their way independently (O'Malley et al., 2018).

Interestingly, the shape or configuration of the residential care home also matters. L-shaped layouts compared to H- or square-shaped layouts seem to decrease disorientation (Elmståhl et al., 1997). Subsequently, residents were better at finding their way in buildings with a straight circulation system with no change in direction, for example, an I-shaped corridor (Marquardt & Schmieg, 2009). Finally, small-scale residences with simple layouts and clear visual access to both close and distant areas seem to help reduce spatial disorientation (e.g., Marquardt & Schmieg, 2009). In summary, the simpler, the smaller, and more accessible the layout and design of a residential care home, the easier it is for older residents to find their way and feel comfortable and satisfied with the residential care home.

As for the usage of signage, conceived as an environmental cue (Passini et al., 2000), signs, pictograms, and decorations are useful in residential care homes because they support spatial planning and decision-making for successful wayfinding (Marquardt, 2011; O'Malley et al., 2018). To increase their effectiveness, signage and environmental cues should be placed near major turning points or intersections (Carpman & Grant, 2002) and should include not only text but also pictorial information to contrast possible difficulties in reading comprehension in PwD (Klimova & Kuca, 2016). Even personal items placed in or near rooms can also act as signposts. Decorating rooms and buildings with personal objects, furniture, photographs, and names can help older people easily identify their rooms (typically located in long, non-functional corridors). Personal home items could thus provide both a reference point for the elderly by facilitating their orientation and also give a homelike character, which has also been seen to improve functioning, autonomy, and interactions in residential care homes (Chaudhury et al., 2018).

Alongside the layout and signage, it is important to consider the internal organization of spaces (Abu-Obeid, 1998). Indeed, identifying places represents one of the major challenges for PwD (Passini et al., 2000), who need to recognize the floor where they reside, their own room, and common areas such as the dining room or the entrance hall. By creating visually distinct elements with different sizes, shapes, architectural styles, and colours, residents are less likely to become lost or confused. Visual differentiation of the environment improves navigability and supports wayfinding and navigational behaviours (e.g., O'Malley et al., 2018). Distinguishing rooms from each other or daytime areas from bedrooms can be done by differentiating furniture, decorations, walls, and door colours.

Besides navigability, there are other features of the building that can influence wayfinding and orientation within it. First, ensuring good quality and quantity of light is important for older adults' circadian rhythm, perception, and motion. Moreover, a recent review found that the presence of light inside the building is also a predictor of older adults' orientation

(Goudriaan et al., 2021). Similarly, good acoustic quality (low noise) can also facilitate orientation in residential care homes (Marquardt et al., 2014).

In summary, layout, signage, visual differentiation, adequate light, and noise reduction can play a key role in a resident's ability to move independently and orient to the environment from a structural (i.e., layout), visual (i.e., differentiation), and semantic (i.e., signage) point of view.

Assessing and improving navigability of residential care homes

The quality assessment of a long-term care facility physical environment, also in terms of navigability, would allow professionals and stakeholders to plan architectural design solutions that support users' experiences of their accommodations and, therefore, their autonomy and wellbeing, according to economic and regulation constraints. There are several tools available for the assessment of the quality of the physical environment of healthcare facilities for PwD, such as the EVOLVE design toolkit or the Environmental Audit Tool (see Calkins et al., 2022; Elf et al., 2017; O'Malley et al., 2018). In general, these instruments are focused on environmental characteristics different from navigability or, at best, comprise a few items specifically detecting navigability issues (O'Malley et al., 2018). For example, the Professional Environmental Assessment Protocol (Lawton et al., 2000) includes items that allow trained professionals to assess the presence of aids for orientation in special care units for PwD.

Recently, the Residential Care Home Navigability scale (Miola et al., 2023) has been purposely developed for the assessment of navigability in residential care homes. The scale has been designed to detect respondents' experience of layout complexity, differentiation of visual, spatial, and design features, signage systems of residential care homes, and was conceived to be administered not only to older residents but also to their informal caregivers and members of the care home's staff. It has been validated by a sample of residents (both without cognitive impairments and in the mild dementia stage), informal caregivers, and staff members from 13 Italian residential care homes. Respondents' positive evaluations of the navigability of their accommodation-workplace was associated with a greater perceived sense of direction. Layout and signage contributed to a better experience of sense of direction, especially among older residents.

Alongside the paucity of instruments for the assessment of navigability of residential care homes, guidelines for practitioners towards interventions for a supportive environment in terms of navigability remain vague. Environmental interventions usually occur when the facility is already constructed. Environmental interventions specifically targeting spatial orientation and wayfinding could thus focus, rather than on modifying the architectural layout, on incorporating appropriate signage and useful, salient landmarks as well as on improving visual differentiation of the environment (Miola et al., 2023; Wiener & Pazzaglia, 2021). Nonetheless, wayfinding and spatial orientation are usually not considered an independent, key design principle. Solutions such as adapting signage, colours, lighting, or furniture to the needs of PwD usually fall within broader design principles of supporting movement, optimizing stimulation, and ensuring accessibility.

Concluding remarks and further directions

Wayfinding represents a crucial skill for individual's everyday autonomy and wellbeing across the entire lifespan. A deterioration in such abilities is not only common with increasing age and among PwD, but also among the early markers of cognitive impairment.

With the increasing aging of the population, and therefore of the number of people who may live in residential care homes, understanding the interplay between vulnerabilities in wayfinding behaviours and the environment becomes paramount. Indeed, the physical environment, with its architectural and design features, could make a difference towards allowing PwD living in such complex indoor environments to maintain their autonomy. Environmental features related to layout, signage, visual differentiation could improve the navigability of residential care homes and, thus, minimize spatial disorientation and wayfinding problems among PwD.

Nonetheless, more research, adopting a mixed-method, multidisciplinary and longitudinal approach, is warranted to further identify nuanced and flexible environmental solutions capable of supporting navigability in PwD considering their different individual profiles and the changing states of the disorder. To what extent the use of emerging assistive technology would be integrated to aid orientation and wayfinding in long-term care facilities also warrants further investigation. Alongside the importance of considering the PwD point of view and experiences, the perspectives of visitors, such as family caregivers who could be older adults too, as well as staff members still need to be further accounted. The ease of navigating within long-term care facilities could indeed impact the quality of care and assistance provided by formal and informal caregivers and, thus, health and wellbeing outcomes of PwD. For example, staff should move easily within the facility to perform their job in the best and quick way possible, moreover, if the older residents are more autonomous in wayfinding, the staff spend less time to accompany or assist the older adults in travelling and reaching destinations within the building.

An interdisciplinary approach and the joint effort of different disciplines, including environmental psychology, would also better translate experimental evidence into reliable assessment tools, as well as design guidelines and practical solutions, available for practitioners and stakeholders to prompt the environmental quality of long-term care facilities also in terms of navigability. Psychologists, care providers, architects, and designers, bringing together their expertise in aging and environmental psychology with regards to the environmental characteristics of buildings, should work in synergy to design buildings or develop environmental interventions in existing structures to provide an environment functional and supportive for its users.

In conclusion, a well-designed and supportive environment represents one of the key components of care for PwD. Finding ways to express the therapeutic potential of the environment in the context of residential care homes, also when crucial skills as wayfinding and navigation are concerned, would improve the lives of PwD and those who take care of them.

In-depth box

- Theoretical models of indoor wayfinding according to the cognitive and environmental psychology perspectives are presented.
- Age- and disease-related impairments in wayfinding behaviours are discussed, highlighting the impact of relocation in new long-term living accommodation for people with dementia's autonomy and wellbeing.
- Evidence of environmental solutions to improve residential care homes' navigability and its factors (layout, signage, and visual differentiation) and to support older residents with dementia orientation and wayfinding are summarized according to recent commentaries or literature reviews.
- The availability of instruments for the assessment of navigability in long-term care facilities as well as guidelines for improving it are discussed.

References

Abu-Obeid, N. (1998). Abstract and scenographic imagery: The effect of environmental form on wayfinding. *Journal of Environmental Psychology, 18*, 159–173. https://doi.org/10.1006/jevp.1998.0082

Baskaya, A., Wilson, C., & Özcan, Y. Z. (2004). Wayfinding in an unfamiliar environment: Different spatial settings of two polyclinics. *Environment and Behavior, 36*, 839–867. https://doi.org/10.1177/0013916504265445

Böckerman, P., Johansson, E., & Saarni, S. I. (2012). Institutionalisation and subjective wellbeing for old-age individuals: Is life really miserable in care homes? *Ageing & Society, 32*, 1176–1192. https://doi.org/10.1017/S0144686X1100081X

Brownie, S., Horstmanshof, L., & Garbutt, R. (2014). Factors that impact residents' transition and psychological adjustment to long-term aged care: A systematic literature review. *International Journal of Nursing Studies, 51*, 1654–1666. https://doi.org/10.1016/j.ijnurstu.2014.04.011

Calkins, M. P., Kaup, M. L., & Abushousheh, A. M. (2022). Evaluation of environmental assessment tools for settings for individuals living with dementia. *Alzheimer's & Dementia: Translational Research & Clinical Interventions, 8*, e12353. https://doi.org/10.1002/trc2.12353

Carbone, E., Gardini, S., Pastore, M., Piras, F., Vincenzi, M., & Borella, E. (2021a). Cognitive stimulation therapy for older adults with mild-to-moderate dementia in Italy: Effects on cognitive functioning, and on emotional and neuropsychiatric symptoms. *The Journals of Gerontology: Series B, 76*, 1700–1710. https://doi.org/10.1093/geronb/gbab007

Carbone, E., Meneghetti, C., & Borella, E. (2021b). Supporting route learning in older adults: The role of imagery strategy. *Aging & Mental Health, 25*, 1564–1571. https://doi.org/10.1080/13607863.2020.1727844

Carlson, L. A., Hölscher, C., Shipley, T. F., & Dalton, R. C. (2010) Getting lost in buildings. *Current Directions in Psychological Science, 19*, 284–289. https://doi.org/10. 1177/0963721410383243

Carpman, J. R., & Grant, M. A. (2002). Wayfinding: A broad view. In R. B. Bechtel & A. Churchman (Eds.), *Handbook of environmental psychology* (pp. 427–442). Wiley.

Castle, N. G. (2001). Relocation of the elderly. *Medical Care Research and Review, 58*, 291–333. https://doi.org/10.1177/107755870105800302

Chaudhury, H., Cooke, H. A., Cowie, H., & Razaghi, L. (2018). The influence of the physical environment on residents with dementia in long-term care settings: A review of the empirical literature. *The Gerontologist, 58*, e325–e337. https://doi.org/10.1093/geront/gnw259

Coughlan, G., Coutrot, A., Khondoker, M., Minihane, A.M., Spiers, H., & Hornberger, M. (2019). Toward personalized cognitive diagnostics of at-genetic-risk Alzheimer's disease. *Proceedings of the National Academy of Sciences, 116*, 9285–9292.

Devlin, A. S. (2014). Wayfinding in healthcare facilities: Contributions from environmental psychology. *Behavioral Sciences, 4*, 423–436. https://doi.org/10.3390/bs4040423

Elf, M., Nordin, S., Wijk, H., & Mckee, K.J. (2017). A systematic review of the psychometric properties of instruments for assessing the quality of the physical environment in healthcare. *Journal of Advanced Nursing, 73*, 2796–2816. https://doi.org/10.1111/jan.13281

Elmståhl, S., Annerstedt, L., & Ahlund, O. (1997). How should a group living unit for demented elderly be designed to decrease psychiatric symptoms? *Alzheimer Disease and Associated Disorders, 11*(1), 47–52. https://doi.org/10.1097/00002093-199703000-00008

Golledge, R. G. (1987). Environmental cognition. In: D. Stokols & I. Altman (Eds.), *Handbook of environmental psychology* (pp. 131–174). Wiley.

Goudriaan, I., Van Boekel, L. C., Verbiest, M. E., Van Hoof, J., & Luijkx, K. G. (2021). Dementia enlightened?! A systematic literature review of the influence of indoor environmental light on the health of older persons with dementia in long-term care facilities. *Clinical Interventions in Aging, 16*, 909–937. https://doi.org/10.2147/CIA.S297865

Harris, M. A., & Wolbers, T. (2014). How age-related strategy switching deficits affect wayfinding in complex environments. *Neurobiology of Aging, 35*, 1095–1102. https://doi.org/10.1016/j.neurobiolaging. 2013.10.086

Jamshidi, S., Ensafi, M., & Pati, D. (2020). Wayfinding in interior environments: An integrative review. *Frontiers in Psychology, 11*, 549628. https://doi.org/10.3389/fpsyg.2020.549628

Klencklen, G., Després, O., & Dufour, A. (2012). What do we know about aging and spatial cognition? Reviews and perspectives. *Ageing Research Reviews, 11*, 123–135. https://doi.org/10.1016/j.arr.2011.10.001

Klimova, B., & Kuca, K. (2016) Speech and language impairments in dementia. *Journal of Applied Biomedicine, 14*, 97–103. https://doi.org/10.1016/j.jab. 2016.02.002

Kunz, L., Schröder, T. N., Lee, H., Montag, C., Lachmann, B., Sariyska, R., & Fell, J. (2015). Reduced grid-cell-like representations in adults at genetic risk for Alzheimer's disease. *Science, 350*, 430–433. https://doi.org/10.1126/science.aac8128

Lawton, M. P. (1977). The impact of environment on ageing and behaviour. In: K. W. Schaie & J. E. Birren (Eds.). *Handbook of physiology of ageing* (pp. 276–301). Van Nostrand Reinhold.

Lawton, M. P., Weisman, G. D., Sloane, P., Norris-Baker, C., Calkins, M., & Zimmerman, S. I. (2000). Professional environmental assessment procedure for special care units for elders with dementing illness and its relationship to the therapeutic environment screening schedule. *Alzheimer Disease & Associated Disorders, 14*, 28–38.

Lester, A. W., Moffat, S. D., Wiener, J. M., Barnes, C. A., & Wolbers, T. (2017). The aging navigational system. *Neuron, 95*, 1019–1035. https://doi. org/10.1016/j. neuron.2017.06.037

Marquardt, G. (2011). Wayfinding for people with dementia: A review of the role of architectural design. *HERD: Health Environments Research & Design Journal, 4*, 75–90. https://doi.org/10.1177/193758671100400207

Marquardt, G., Bueter, K., & Motzek, T. (2014). Impact of the design of the built environment on people with dementia: An evidence-based review. *HERD: Health Environments Research & Design Journal, 8*, 127–157.

Marquardt, G., & Schmieg, P. (2009). Dementia-friendly architecture: Environments that facilitate wayfinding in nursing homes. *American Journal of Alzheimer's Disease & Other Dementias, 24*, 333–340. https://doi.org/10.1177/1533317509334959

Meneghetti, C., Borella, E., Carbone, E., Martinelli, M., & De Beni, R. (2016). Environment learning using descriptions or navigation: The involvement of working memory in young and older adults. *British Journal of Psychology, 107*, 259–280. https://doi.org/10.1111/bjop.12145

Miola, L., Carbone, E., Toffalini, E., & Pazzaglia, F. (2023). Navigability of residential care homes from residents', family members', and staff's points of view: The residential care home navigability scale. *The Gerontologist, 63*, 1419–1427. https://doi.org/10.1093/geront/gnad029

Mitolo, M., Borella, E., Meneghetti, C., Carbone, E., & Pazzaglia, F. (2017). How to enhance route learning and visuo-spatial working memory in aging: A training for residential care home residents. *Aging & Mental Health, 21*, 562–570. https://doi. org/10.1080/13607863.2015.1132673

Mitolo, M., Gardini, S., Fasano, F., Crisi, G., Pelosi, A., Pazzaglia, F., & Caffarra, P. (2013). Visuospatial memory and neuroimaging correlates in mild cognitive impairment. *Journal of Alzheimer's Disease, 35*, 75–90. https://doi.org/10.3233/JAD-121288

O'Malley, M., Innes, A., Muir, S., & Wiener, J. M. (2018). 'All the corridors are the same': A qualitative study of the orientation experiences and design preferences of UK older adults living in a communal retirement development. *Ageing & Society, 38*, 1791–1816. https://doi.org/10.1017/S0144686X17000277

Passini, R., Pigot, H., Rainville, C., & Tétreault, M. H. (2000). Wayfinding in a nursing home for advanced dementia of the Alzheimer's type. *Environment and Behavior, 32*, 684–710. https://doi.org/10.1177/0013916002197274

Ryman, F. V., Erisman, J. C., Darvey, L. M., Osborne, J., Swartsenburg, E., & Syurina, E. V. (2019). Health effects of the relocation of patients with dementia: A scoping review to inform medical and policy decision-making. *The Gerontologist, 59*, e674-e682. https://doi.org/10.1093/geront/gny031

Salimi, S., Irish, M., Foxe, D., Hodges, J. R., Piguet, O., & Burrell, J. R. (2018). Can visuospatial measures improve the diagnosis of Alzheimer's disease? *Alzheimer's & Dementia: Diagnosis, Assessment & Disease Monitoring, 10*, 66–74. https://doi.org/10.1016/j.dadm.2017.10.004

Tao, Y., Gou, Z., Lau, S. S. Y., Lu, Y., & Fu, J. (2018). Legibility of floor plans and wayfinding satisfaction of residents in Care and Attention homes in Hong Kong. *Australasian Journal on Ageing, 37*, E139–E143. https://doi.org/10.1111/ajag.12574

Tolman, E. C. (1948). Cognitive maps in rats and men. *Psychological Review, 55*, 189–208. https://doi.org/10.1037/h0061626

van der Ham, I. J., Claessen, M. H., Evers, A. W., & van der Kuil, M. N. (2020). Large-scale assessment of human navigation ability across the lifespan. *Scientific Reports, 10*, 3299. https://doi.org/10.1038/s41598-020-60302-0

Wiener, J. M., & Pazzaglia, F. (2021). Ageing-and dementia-friendly design: Theory and evidence from cognitive psychology, neuropsychology and environmental psychology can contribute to design guidelines that minimise spatial disorientation. *Cognitive Processing, 22*, 715–730. https://doi.org/10.1007/s10339-021-01031-8

Green care farms and other innovative settings

Hilde Verbeek, Ingeborg Pedersen,
Bram de Boer and Simone de Bruin

The environment plays a crucial role to support people living with dementia in their daily functioning, especially when the disease progresses, and 24-hour care is needed. There is growing recognition that traditional care models fall short for people with dementia and their family caregivers as they are not effective in supporting everyday functioning and may even be harmful (Eckermann et al., 2019). This has led to a call for new dementia care approaches which urgently need alternative care environments, using enabling environmental design to promote health and well-being of people living with dementia. In response, innovations in long-term dementia care are taking place both in the community and in residential care, one of which is the care concept called *care farming*.

First, the chapter discusses care farming and its impact. Second, the general theoretical underpinnings of the care farm environment will be explored using an environmental framework (De Boer et al., 2021a). Third, other innovative care settings will be presented and compared using this framework.

Care farming and its impact on well-being

Care farming is an intervention for promoting health and well-being through the use of a farm environment as the central element and has been used for various client groups (Hassink et al., 2010). Care farms serving people living with dementia either provide adult day services (ADSs) during weekdays, or 24-hour care as an alternative for regular nursing homes. Additionally, there is a small number of care farms providing evening or weekend services to people with dementia or respite services to family caregivers (De Bruin et al., 2010). Care farming has different representations and varies both between and within countries. They generally have some degree of commercial farming (i.e. crops, livestock, and woodland) combined with health, social and/or educational care services. There is great variation among care farms regarding the ratio between farming and these services and the types of farming activities (e.g. dairy farm, industrial livestock farm, mixed farm, forestry). Farms can have conventional agricultural production, while others

DOI: 10.4324/9781003416241-22

are primarily care providers (Hassink et al., 2012). Many farmers and staff members have an education in agriculture, health care, and/or social care (e.g. social workers, registered nurses, nurse assistants, nurse aides, occupational therapists, educational staff). Care farms often collaborate with and/or hire staff of regular care settings or could be organised as a part of the municipal care service. Volunteers to assist with the services are common (Hassink et al., 2012; Ibsen et al., 2018).

The Netherlands and Norway are seen as front-runners in providing and researching care at care farms, with 1250 in the Netherlands and 400 registered and an unknown number of unregistered care farms in Norway (De Bruin et al., 2020). Gradually, the concept of care farming is being implemented in other countries, although exact numbers are often unknown. Current estimations indicate: Austria (n=600), Belgium (n=670), France (n=900), Ireland (n=100), Italy (n=675), South Korea (n=30), Switzerland (n=1000), United Kingdom (n=230), and no estimations available for Japan, Poland and the USA (De Bruin et al., 2021b; Garcia-Llorente et al., 2018; Hassink et al., 2020; Haubenhofer et al., 2010; Yewon Chu, personal communication).

Several studies have explored the impact of care farms on people living with dementia, both for participants of ADSs at farms and residents of farms as nursing homes. These studies showed that people living with dementia spent more time outdoors, were more physically active and were more engaged in everyday and meaningful activities, compared with their counterparts in regular care institutions (e.g. De Boer et al., 2017; De Bruin et al., 2009; Garshol et al., 2020). These everyday activities, occurred naturally, and included a wide range of domestic, farm and leisure activities such as folding laundry, preparing meals, weeding the soil, watering the plants, walking the dog, feeding animals, sweeping the lawn, fixing broken furniture/tools, getting wood for the fireplace, and raking or shoveling snow (De Bruin et al., 2009; Ellingsen-Dalskau et al., 2021). As such, care farms support contact with nature and animals, which are both a source for rest and activity (De Bruin et al., 2021; Pedersen et al., 2022). Because of the wide range of activities and locations, people living with dementia and their family caregivers experienced freedom of movement and freedom of choice at farms regarding how and where they would spend their days (De Boer et al., 2019; Ibsen et al., 2018). This can facilitate feelings of autonomy and meaning in life, as people living with dementia still have the opportunity to contribute to the life at the farm (De Bruin et al., 2021; Ibsen et al., 2021).

Care farms positively influence the social health of people living with dementia (Dröes et al., 2017), as the social context of the farm resembles a family-like structure and encourages social participation of people with dementia (De Bruin et al., 2021). Likewise, research showed that people living with dementia had more social interactions at farms than in regular care institutions (De Boer et al., 2017; Finnanger Garshol et al., 2022).

Interactions took place between people with dementia, with family, friends, staff, volunteers but also with people from outside the farm, such as school children visiting the farm and people living in the community (De Bruin et al., 2021). The social interactions were positively associated with the people with dementia's emotional well-being (Finnanger Garshol et al., 2022). They further felt they collaborated closely with staff (Ellingsen-Dalskau et al., 2021; Myren et al., 2017). The homelike atmosphere and supportive social relationships could be the reason why people with dementia describe a sense of community, identity, and belonging (Ibsen & Erikson, 2021; Sudmann & Børsheim, 2017).

Furthermore, research suggests that care farms support structure, healthy eating, and a sense of meaning in life. Participants and their family caregivers experienced less stigmatising because of dementia, since the care farm environment is a homelike non-institutional kind of place. Instead, people living with dementia feel and are treated as a volunteer or employee rather than a patient with cognitive and functional impairments. People living with dementia additionally feel recognised, understood, and seen as people who can deliver a meaningful contribution (De Bruin et al., 2021; Ibsen & Eriksen, 2021; Sudmann & Børsheim, 2017). In addition, care farms promote respite, more personal time, and fewer feelings of guilt among family caregivers. Family caregivers indicated that care farms provide care tailored to the individual needs of people with dementia (De Boer et al., 2019).

Anecdotal evidence suggests that only few people living with dementia are from ethnic minority groups in farm-based long-term care (De Bruin, 2021). They experience limited access to health and social care services, and as such make less frequent use of these services (Duran et al., 2022). An exploratory study of Windesheim University of Applied Sciences in the Netherlands among health and social care professionals, family caregivers, and people living with dementia from ethnic minority groups revealed that care farms may be an attractive form of care (De Bruin, 2021). Interviews showed that care farms corresponded with life habits and preferences of several people from minority groups as they were familiar with farm-based activities such as taking care of animals and growing crops. Furthermore, the hands-on approach of farms provides more opportunities for activity engagement. This does not require extensive language skills as opposed to regular care, with many activities requiring Dutch language skills (e.g., reading the newspaper or word games). Finally, care farms provide space and opportunities for relaxation and finding peace. Part of the migrants are refugees, and many of these have experienced trauma (Alzheimer Europe, 2018). Contact with nature and spending time in a natural environment may reduce feelings of stress and anger, restore mental fatigue, reduce symptoms of post-traumatic stress disorder, and increase feelings of happiness and overall well-being (Gorman & Cacciatore, 2017; Greenleaf & Roessger, 2017; Varning Poulsen, 2017; Varning Poulsen et al., 2016).

Care environment framework

Care farms have radically redesigned the long-term care environment for people living with dementia. Using a co-creation method involving older people, their families, staff, management, architects, and designers, we developed a framework to conceptualise potential environmental working mechanisms (De Boer et al., 2021). It identifies three important components that impact the daily life of people living with dementia:

1 *Physical environment.* This includes all physical aspects in the built environment, such as interior design, outdoor spaces (e.g., gardens), lay-out, and sensory elements. Care farms have a small-scale character breathing out a home-like and familiar atmosphere, which makes people with dementia feel safe and comfortable (Ellingsen-Dalskau & Pedersen, 2022; Myren et al., 2017). People living with dementia have free access to various indoor (e.g. kitchen, living room, work shed) and outdoor environments (e.g. garden, farm yard, stable, green house). They are exposed to normal daily life stimuli and the physical environment stimulates the senses through familiar odours (e.g. hay, silage, food that is being prepared), sounds (e.g. tractors, animals), touch (e.g. animals, soils), and tastes (e.g. fresh fruits and vegetables) (De Bruin et al., 2010; Rosteius et al., 2022). The large diversity of activities provides freedom choice for people living with dementia ample opportunities for staff to tailor activities to people with dementia's skills, interest, and needs (Ellingsen-Dalskau & Pedersen, 2022).

2 *Social environment.* This entails all interactions with others in the environment, including older people, caregivers, and the broader community. Care farm staff use the environment to facilitate an inclusive atmosphere that stimulate mutual connections between people living with dementia and create a community (Rosteius et al., 2022). The closeness and social interaction are a result of the farmer tailoring activities in a way that make all the attendees feel included and able to participate (Ellingsen-Dalskau & Pedersen, 2022). The social environment also builds on the interaction between people with dementia and staff, family and friends. Moreover, some farms have a shop, a restaurant, or freely distribute fruits and vegetables to people in the community, which results in different kinds of people visiting the farm (e.g. children, local entrepreneurs, tourists). As such, care farms are also connected to the wider community and social context in the farm is situated (De Bruin et al., 2021).

3 *Organisational environment.* This reflects the organisation's vision guiding how dementia care is being organised and how the organisational culture is being perceived (e.g., values, expectations, attitudes that guide behaviour that guide staff's behaviour). The organisation's vision reflects how the physical and social environments are being designed and utilised with the farmer and staff as the catalyst. Important elements aspects of farms

are person-centred approach, emphasis on people's abilities (in contrast to their disabilities), autonomy, dignity, and respect for someone's lifestyle, habits, and preferences. The farmer propagates this vision and employs staff and volunteers that have the competences to carry out this vision, e.g., person-centred working, flexibility, creativity, progressive mindset, and willingness to learn and change (Buist et al., 2018; De Boer et al., 2021; Ellingsen-Dalskau & Pedersen 2022).

An ethnographic study, where researchers lived at a care farm in the Netherlands and conducted 28 days of participating observations with residents, family caregivers, and staff revealed four themes as crucial during daily life on care farms: stimulating the senses, engaging in purposeful activities, sharing responsibilities, and creating a community in a new home (Rosteius et al., 2022). To put these topics into practice, the physical, social and organisational environment were highly interrelated. Purposeful design of physical spaces encouraged and facilitated meaningful in-/outdoor activities and social encounters. The leadership and staff's competencies supported the use of the physical environment by aligning processes and transporting the vision. Collaboration and creating a home-like atmosphere by including residents in household- and farm chores characterised the social environment. This community-building led to more meaningful activities and social interaction. Care farm studies show a central role for management in paving the way for a new form of care delivery for people living with dementia (De Bruin et al., 2020; Rosteius et al., 2022).

Innovative small-scale, homelike care environments

As leaders shape the three environments, the organisation influences the design of the physical environment and the actions taking place within it. This provides opportunities for regular care, as these environmental elements of care farms could be implemented in a variety of care settings (Buist et al., 2018). Several other small-scale, homelike care environments have been developed that have radically altered the long-term care environment. To support a person-centred long-term care, these environments look beyond the disability of people living with dementia and focus on their remaining capacities, aiming to enable and preserve gains and positive outcomes.

Small-scale, homelike care environments have been developed in Sweden and the Netherlands in the 80s and 90s (Verbeek et al., 2009). In the Netherlands, the number has risen quickly in the period 2005–2015, partly due to governmental encouragement. Comparable models have been developed in the USA (Green Houses, e.g. Kane et al., 2007) and Germany (Shared Housing Arrangements, e.g. Wolf-Ostermann et al., 2014). All models aim to support residents' autonomy by fostering normalised daily activities, such as doing laundry or cooking, minimising rigid routines, and enabling residents to live their life as normal as possible. Choice and preserving one's identity are key and groups are small (i.e. between 6 and 10 residents per group), allowing staff to form a household with residents and family. Furthermore, staff have integrated tasks, meaning that they are not only responsible for personal and medical care, but also do activities and do household chores (Verbeek et al., 2009). The physical environment resembles an archetypical home. Research into effectiveness has mostly focused on residents, in particular in relation to quality of life and health-related outcomes with mixed results. There seems evidence for a better physical functioning in comparison with traditional nursing homes and a higher satisfaction with care (Ausserhofer et al., 2016). Furthermore, differences were found for staff's job characteristics, with more perceived job autonomy, social support and less perceived demands (e.g., Adams et al., 2017; Willemse et al., 2014). No effect for family- or staff related outcomes were identified (Ausserhofer et al., 2016).

The Dementia Village is another model that aims to create a homelike atmosphere, focusing on autonomy but is not small-scaled. Originated from the Netherlands (de Hogeweyk), dementia villages have now been developed in Denmark, Germany and France, often located in mid-sized towns (e.g., Peoples et al., 2020). They create an environment that enables residents to live as normally as possible, while still feeling part of a local community. The village is designed to resemble a familiar environment with landmarks such as a high street, town square, supermarket, activity centre, connecting paths between residences, and gardens. First indications showed that family of people living with dementia and staff were committed to creating and maintaining a meaningful everyday life for the residents, but also revealed different understandings of when, where, and how this could be understood and best be achieved (Peoples et al., 2020). Furthermore, it was uncertain what the added value could be for people living with advanced dementia.

A wide range of international examples show that innovative and inclusive care environments can be developed in both rural and urbanised areas (e.g., Fleming et al., 2020). They are embedded within the local community to foster inclusion, equity, and dignity for residents. A Dutch housing association (Habion) has developed a specific method to include the local community in the co-creation process of long-term care environments, called the Røring method (van Hoof et al., 2020). The Liv Inn project (liv-inn.nl) is an example in which they have implemented it in practice. A former assisted living facility was redesigned into a new setting for a variety of groups, including older people living with dementia and younger persons. The redesign developed gradually in interaction with residents and the local community (Verbeek et al., 2021). Values including independence, security and their self-identity, choice and memories are essential and residents are in charge to oversee their care and how the building should be designed. The Røring method facilitates interested actors and residents to be motivated and enthusiastic, while maintaining inclusivity in its nature.

Future directions

There is an urgent need for the development and design of inclusive care environments in long-term care, that increase older persons' agency, support their human rights, and enables person-centred care (Verbeek et al., 2021). These can be either home- or community-based, exploring concepts such as caring neighbourhoods or vital communities, but also include collective living arrangements and residential environments such as nursing homes. More evidence-based knowledge is highly needed to develop innovative housing with care strategies, interventions and programs, preventing ageism, and incorporating intergenerational approaches to explore opportunities to create a new, neighbourhood perspective to long-term care and being inclusive to all. This requires different care competencies of staff, focusing on enhancing capacity and increasing functional abilities (De Boer et al., 2021). Furthermore, the use of technology (e.g., wearables, sensors) and artificial intelligence in environmental design may help enable more freedom and support autonomy of people living with dementia. In this way, inclusive living becomes available for all. Finally, more knowledge is needed regarding the social capital long-term care environments may have on the local community. This included the emergence of citizen initiatives, where older persons themselves develop housing with care initiatives.

In-depth box

- The chapter used a human-rights based perspective on environmental design, i.e. promoting dignity, liberty and security, enjoying good health and continue participation in society aiming inclusivity to all (regardless someone's gender, age, social-economic position, ethnic or religious background, sexuality).
- Many primary studies described in this chapter used a Living Lab approach building on long-lasting relationships with people living with dementia, their caregivers, and staff on locations. This facilitated building individual, trusting relationships, which ultimately are the key to understanding contexts, culture, and mechanisms of change.
- Environmental design in this chapter emphasises the co-creation and results from an important interplay between physical, social, and organisational aspects of the care environment.

References

Alzheimer Europe. (2018). *The development of intercultural care and support for people with dementia from minority ethnic groups.* https://www.alzheimer-europe. org/sites/default/files/alzheimer_europe_ethics_report_2018.pdf

Adams, J., Verbeek, H., & Zwakhalen, S. M. G. (2017). The impact of organizational innovations in nursing homes on staff perceptions: a secondary data analysis. *Journal of Nursing Scholarship*, 49(1), 54–62. https://doi.org/10.1111/jnu.12271

Ausserhofer, D., Deschodt, M., De Geest, S., van Achterberg, T., Meyer, G., Verbeek, H., Sjetne, I. S., Malinowska-Lipień, I., Griffiths, P., Schlüter, W., Ellen, M., & Engberg, S. (2016). "There's no place like home": a scoping review on the impact of homelike residential care models on resident-, family-, and staff-related outcomes. *Journal of the American Medical Directors Association*, *17*(8), 685–693. https://doi.org/10.1016/j.jamda.2016.03.009

Buist, Y., Verbeek, H., de Boer, B., & de Bruin, S.R. (2018). Innovating dementia care; Implementing characteristics of green care farms in other long-term care settings. *International Psychogeriatrics*, *30*(7), 1057–1068. https://doi.org/10.1017/S1041610217002848

De Boer, B., Bozdemir, B., Jansen, J., Hermans, M., Hamers, J.P.H., & Verbeek, H. (2021a). The homestead: developing a conceptual framework through co-creation for innovating long-term dementia care environments. *International Journal of Environmental Research and Public Health*, *18*(1), 57. https://doi.org/10.3390/ijerph18010057

De Boer, B., Buist, Y., De Bruin, S., Backhaus, R., & Verbeek, H. (2021b). Working at green care farms and other innovative small-scale long-term dementia care facilities requires different competencies of care staff. *International Journal of Environmental Research and Public Health*, *18*(20), 10747. https://doi.org/10.3390/ijerph182010747

De Boer, B., Hamers, J.P.H., Zwakhalen, S.M.G, Tan, F. E., Beerens, H.C., & Verbeek, H. (2017). Green care farms as innovative nursing homes, promoting activities and social interaction for people with dementia. *Journal of the American Medical Directors Association*, *18*(1), 40–46. https://doi.org/10.1016/j.jamda.2016.10.013

De Boer, B., Verbeek, H., Zwakhalen, S.M.G., & Hamers, J.P.H. (2019). Experiences of family caregivers in green care farms and other nursing home environments for people with dementia: a qualitative study. *BMC Geriatrics*, *19*(1), 149. https://doi.org/10.1186/s12877-019-1163-6

De Bruin, S.R. (2021). *Geen beter leven dan een goed leven (No better life than a good life)*. Zwolle: Windesheim University of Applied Sciences, Department of Health and Well-being.

De Bruin, S.R., Buist, Y., Hassink, J., & Vaandrager, L. (2021a). "I want to make myself useful": the value of nature-based adult day services in urban areas for people with dementia and their family carers. *Ageing & Society*, *41*(3), 582–604. https://doi.org/10.1017/S0144686X19001168

De Bruin, S.R, Hassink, J., Vaandrager, L., De Boer, B., Verbeek, H., & Pedersen, I., Grindal, G., Patil, L.H., & Ellingsen-Dalskau, S.E. (2021b). Care farms: a health-promoting context for a wide range of client groups. In E. Brymer, M. Rogerson, & J. Barton (Eds.), *Nature and health; physical activity in nature* (pp. 177–190). New York/Oxon: Routledge.

De Bruin, S.R., Oosting, S.J., Enders-Slegers, M.J., van der Zijpp, A.J., & Schols, J.M.G.A. (2010). The concept of green care farms for demented elderly: an integrative framework. *Dementia*, *9*(1), 79–128.

De Bruin, S.R., Oosting, S.J., Kuin, Y., Hoefnagels, E. C. M., Blauw, Y.H., De Groot, L.C.P.G.M., & Schols, J.M.G.A. (2009). Green care farms promote activity among elderly people with dementia. *Journal of Housing for the Elderly*, *23*(4), 368–389. https://doi.org/10.1080/02763890903327275

De Bruin, S.R., Pedersen, I., Eriksen, S., Hassink, J., Vaandrager, L., & Grindal Patil, G. (2020). Care farming for people with dementia; what can healthcare leaders learn from this innovative care concept? *Journal of Healthcare Leadership*, 12, 11–18. https://doi.org/10.2147/JHL.S202988

Dröes, R.M., Chattat, R., Diaz, A., Gove, D., Graff, M., Murphy, K., Verbeek, H., Vernooij-Dassen, M., Clare, L., Johannessen, A., Roes, M., Verhey, F., Charras, K., & the INTERDEM Social Health Taskforce (2017). Social health and dementia: a European consensus on the operationalization of the concept and directions for research and practice. *Aging & Mental Health*, 21(1), 1–14. https://doi.org/10.108 0/13607863.2016.1254596

Duran, G., Uysal-Bozkir, O., Uittenbroek, R., Van Hout, H., & Broese van Groenou, M.I. (2022). *Accessibility of health care experienced by persons with dementia from ethnic minority groups and formal and informal caregivers: a scoping review of European literature.* Dementia. https://doi.org/10.1177/14713012211055307

Eckermann, S., Phillipson, L., & Fleming, R. (2019). Re-design of aged care environments is key to improved care quality and cost-effective reform of aged and health system care. *Applied Health Economics and Health Policy*, 17, 127–130. https:// doi.org/10.1007/s40258-018-0435-1

Ellingsen-Dalskau, L.H., De Boer, B., & Pedersen, I. (2021). Comparing the care environment at farm-based and regular day care for people with dementia in Norway - An observational study. *Health and Social Care in the Community*, 29(2), 506–514. https://doi.org/10.1111/hsc.13113

Ellingsen-Dalskau, L.H., & Pedersen, I. (2022). Turning the ordinary into the extraordinary – Experiences of providing farm-based day care for people with dementia. *Wellbeing, Space and Society*, 3, 100119. https://doi.org/10.1016/j. wss.2022.100119

Finnanger Garshol, B., Ellingsen-Dalskau, L.H., & Pedersen, I. (2020). Physical activity in people with dementia attending farm-based dementia day care – A comparative actigraphy study. *BMC Geriatrics*, 20, 219. https://doi.org/10.1186/ s12877-020-01618-4

Finnanger Garshol, B., Pedersen, I., Patil, G., Eriksen, S., & Ellingsen-Dalskau, L.H. (2022). Emotional well-being in people with dementia – A comparative study of farm-based and regular day care services in Norway. *Health and Social Care in the Community*, 30(5), e1734–e1745. https://doi.org/10.1111/hsc.13601

Fleming, R., Zeisel, J., & Bennet, K. (2020). *World Alzheimer's Report 2020: Design, dignity, dementia: dementia-related design and the built environment. Volume 2: Case Studies.* London, England: Alzheimer's Disease International. https://www. alzint.org/u/WorldAlzheimerReport2020Vol2.pdf

Garcia-Llorente, M., Rubio-Olivar, R., and Gutierrez-Briceno, I. (2018). Farming for life quality and sustainability: a literature review of green care research trends in Europe. *International Journal of Environmental Research and Public Health*, 15(6), 1282.

Gorman, R. & Cacciatore, J. (2017). Cultivating our humanity: A systematic review of care farming & traumatic grief. *Health Place*, 47, 12–21.

Greenleaf A, & Roessger, K. (2017). Effectiveness of care farming on veterans' life satisfaction, optimism, and perceived loneliness. *Journal of Humanistic Counselling*, 56: 86–110.

Hassink, J., Agricola, H., Veen, E., Pijpker, R., De Bruin, S., Van der Meulen, H., & Plug, L.B. (2020). The care farming sector in the Netherlands: a reflection on its developments and promising innovations *Sustainability*, 12(9), 3811. https://doi. org/10.3390/su12093811

Hassink, J., Elings, M., Zweekhorst, M., Van Den Nieuwenhuizen, N., & Smit, A. (2010). Care farms in the Netherlands: attractive empowerment-oriented and strengths-based practices in the community. *Health & Place, 16*(3), 423–430. https://doi.org/10.1016/j.healthplace.2009.10.016

Hassink, J., Hulsink, W., & Grin, J. (2012). Care farms in the Netherlands: an under-explored example of multifunctional agriculture – Toward an empirically grounded, organization-theory-based typology. *Rural Sociology, 77*(4), 569–600. https://doi.org/10.1111/j.1549-0831.2012.00089.x

Haubenhofer, D., Elings, M., Hassink, J., & Hine, R. (2010). The development of green care in Western European countries. *Explore, 6*(2), 106–111.

Ibsen, I., & Eriksen, S. (2021). The experience of attending farm-based day care service from the perspective of people with dementia; a qualitative study. *Dementia, 20*(4), 1356–1374.

Ibsen, T.L., Eriksen, S., & Patil, G.G. (2018). Farm-based day care in Norway – a complementary service for people with dementia. *Journal of Multidisciplinary Healthcare, 11*, 349–358. https://doi.org/10.2147/JMDH.S167135

Kane, R.A., Lum, T.Y., Cutler, L.J., Degenholtz, H.B., & Yu, T.C. (2007). Resident outcomes in small-house nursing homes: a longitudinal evaluation of the initial green house program. *Journal of the American Geriatrics Society, 55*(6), 832–839. https://doi.org/10.1111/j.1532-5415.2007.01169.x

Myren, G.E.S., Enmarker, I.C., Hellzén, O., & Saur, E. (2017). The influence of place on everyday life: observations of persons with dementia in regular day care and at the green care farm. *Health, 9*(2), 261–278. https://doi.org/10.4236/health.2017.92018

Pedersen, I., Ellingsen-Dalskau, L., & Patil, G. (2022). Characteristics of farm-based day care services for people with dementia – mapping the stakeholders' views. *Well-being, Space and Society, 3*, 100073. https://doi.org/10.1016/j.wss.2022.100073

Peoples, H., Pedersen, L.F., & Moestrup, L. (2020). Creating a meaningful everyday life: perceptions of relatives of people with dementia and healthcare professionals in the context of a Danish dementia village. *Dementia, 19*(7), 2314–2331. https://doi.org/10.1177/1471301218820480

Rosteius, K., de Boer, B., Staudacher, S., Schols, J. & Verbeek, H. (2022) How the interrelated physical, social and organizational environment impacts daily life of residents with dementia on a Green Care Farm. *Frontiers in Public Health, 10*, 946962. https://doi.org/10.3389/fpubh.2022.946962

Sudmann, T.T., & Børsheim, I.T. (2017). It's good to be useful': activity provision on green care farms in Norway for people living with dementia. *International Practice Development Journal, 7*(Suppl), 1–14. https://doi.org/10.19043/ipdj.7SP.008

Van Hoof, J., Boerenfijn, P., Beneken genaamd Kolmer, D.M., Marston, H.R., Kazak, J.K., & Verbeek, H. (2020). Environmental design for an ageing population. In A. Phelan & D. O'Shea (Eds.), *Changing horizons in the 21st century: perspectives on ageing* (pp. 268–290). Cambridge Scholars Publishing. https://cambridgescholars.com/product/978-1-5275-4284-6

Varning Poulsen, D. (2017). Nature-based therapy as a treatment for veterans with PTSD: what do we know? *Journal of Public Mental Health, 16*(1): 15–20.

Varning Poulsen, D., Stigsdotter, U., Djernis, D., & Sidenius, U. (2016). Everything just seems much more right in nature: how veterans with post-traumatic stress disorder experience nature-based activities in a forest therapy garden. *Health Psychology Open, 3*(1). https://doi.org/10.1177/2055102916637090

Verbeek, H., Peisah, C., Lima, C.A.M., Rabheru, K., & Ayalon, L. (2021). Human rights to inclusive living and care for older people with mental health conditions. *The American Journal of Geriatric Psychiatry, 29*(10), 1015–1020. https://doi.org/10.1016/j.jagp.2021.05.023

Verbeek, H., Van Rossum, E., Zwakhalen, S.M.G., Kempen, G.I.J.M., & Hamers, J.P.H. (2009). Small, homelike care environments for older people with dementia: a literature review. *International Psychogeriatrics, 21*(2), 252–264. https://doi.org/10.1017/S104161020800820X

Willemse, B.M., Depla, M.F.I.A., Smit, D., & Pot, A.M. (2014). The relationship between small-scale nursing home care for people with dementia and staff's perceived job characteristics. *International Psychogeriatrics, 26*(5), 805–816. https://doi.org/10.1017/S1041610214000015

Wolf-Ostermann, K., Worch, A., Meyer, S., & Gräske, J. (2014). Quality of care and its impact on quality of life for care-dependent persons with dementia in shared-housing arrangements: results of the Berlin WGQual-study. *Applied Nursing Research, 27*(1), 33–40. https://doi.org/10.1016/j.apnr.2013.11.002

Yewon Cho, E., Number of care farms in South Korea (personal communication). 2020.

Selected innovative research projects II

Introduction

This chapter describes two further innovative research projects by early-career researchers (see also Chapter 10, this volume) that add novel perspectives, innovative research methods, and personal reflections on their lessons-learnt to the current discourse of dementia and design.

1 The first contribution, authored by Anne Fahsold and Bernhard Holle, describes lessons-learned when working with an established environmental assessment tool designed to evaluate how dementia-sensitive a built environment is.
2 The second contribution, by Rachel Daly, focuses on identifying critical enabling factors for shared everyday decision-making in care homes.

DOI: 10.4324/9781003416241-23

Project 1

The German Environmental Audit Tool in nursing homes

Anne Fahsold and Bernhard Holle

Dementia & design – what is our perspective?

As health care researchers, our general research focus is on care provision and its structural determinants. In this context, we consider the built environment as a key feature of dementia-specific residential long-term care. When we look at designing for dementia, we are always looking at built environments that have already been built, bearing in mind that: (1) most nursing homes are not built specifically for people with dementia, (2) is necessary to consider the needs of residents without dementia, (3) resident groups and their needs change rapidly.

Regarding the necessity to measure the dementia sensitivity of nursing homes as part of several studies, we were previously confronted with the fact that there was no systematic way to do this in Germany (Palm et al., 2014). Instead of developing a new tool, we decided to adapt an existing and established assessment instrument. We chose the Australian Environmental Audit Tool – High Care (EAT-HC) (Fleming & Bennett, 2015).

Adapting an environmental assessment – who needs to be involved?

Our project to adapt the EAT-HC for the German context consisted of four steps and involved different stakeholder groups, either as experts on the topic or as potential future users (see Figure 17.1).

First, we translated the EAT-HC, consulted scientific experts and practitioners as well as the creators of the EAT-HC. From them, we learned about the underlying concept of the tool – the Key Design Principles (Fahsold, Fleming, et al., 2022). We then tested the new German Environmental Audit Tool (G-EAT) in different nursing homes, including special dementia care units and integrated living units (Fahsold et al., 2022).

We then shared the G-EAT results with the nursing home teams and tried to keep in touch with them regarding whether and how they were using the results to plan environmental adaptations for care provision.

DOI: 10.4324/9781003416241-23

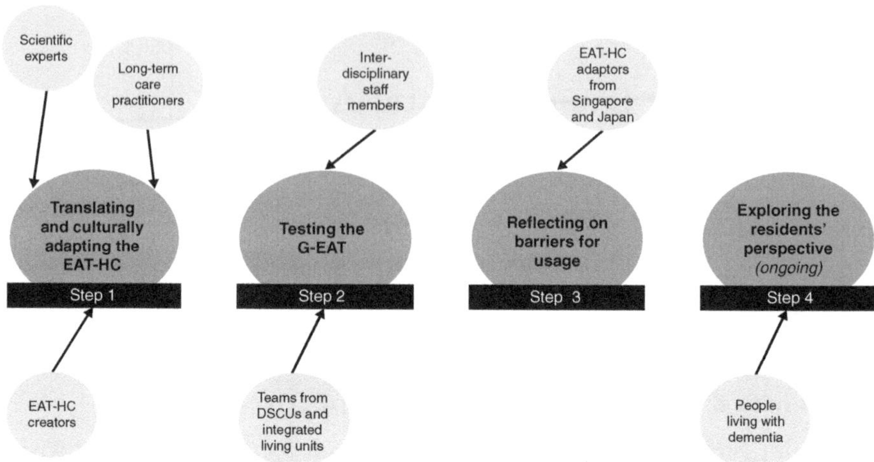

Figure 17.1 Process of adaptation and involvement of stakeholder groups

In doing so, we learnt that there could be many obstacles to using the results of an assessment tool without guidance and reflected on these issues with other EAT-HC adaptors from Singapore and Japan (Fahsold et al., 2023).

As the final step of our project, we wanted to learn about the residents' perspectives on the G-EAT items and scores. However, we then realised that the instrument might benefit from a more holistic involvement of their perspectives on the nursing home environment in general. Hence, we are currently focusing on this in a walking interview study.

Adapting the EAT-HC to the G-EAT – what have we learned?

We have learnt how dementia-specific design is understood by other disciplines. Moreover, we have also learnt about the gap between the idea of dementia-sensitive design in theory and the needs that emerge in practice.

First, the definition of a living unit as a place to live and its structural boundaries may differ between those created by planners, those defined by staff, and those established by residents as a result of their daily living activities. When we do research or a re-design, we need to take this into account.

Second, the involvement of nursing home teams indicated that all staff members are involved in creating dementia-specific environmental features according to the individual needs of residents. In Germany, social workers are particularly important stakeholders as arranging the living environment is a key task.

Finally, our previous and recent experiences are that we need to work on different sets of G-EAT items for practical use and for research. We see that the relevance of some aspects related to the built environment might be less important for residents with dementia in daily life. At the same time, other aspects that are more closely linked to the social environment would be out of the scope for our research purpose.

In-depth box

* To stay with the underlying concept of the EAT-HC and to disseminate it to German practitioners in nursing home care, it was beneficial for us to learn directly from the EAT-HC creators.
* To create a valid and reliable assessment tool for the new cultural context, the involvement of staff from the initial step of translation helped us to include their perspectives.
* To consider that aspects of built environment can differ from those in the literature and our view, the perspective of residents with dementia has been our recent focus.

References

Fahsold, A., Brennan, S., Doan, T., Sun, J., Palm, R., Verbeek, H., & Holle, B. (2023). Adapting the Australian Environmental Assessment Tool-High Care (EAT-HC): Experiences and Practical Implications From Germany, Japan, and Singapore. *HERD*, *16*(1), 287–299. https://doi.org/10.1177/19375867221122936

Fahsold, A., Fleming, R., Verbeek, H., Holle, B., & Palm, R. (2022). German Translation, Linguistic Validation, and Cultural Adaptation of the Environmental Audit Tool—High Care. *HERD: Health Environments Research & Design Journal*, *15*(2), 262–276. https://doi.org/10.1177/19375867211043073

Fahsold, A., Schmüdderich, K., Verbeek, H., Holle, B., & Palm, R. (2022). Feasibility, Interrater Reliability and Internal Consistency of the German Environmental Audit Tool (G-EAT). *International Journal of Environmental Research and Public Health*, *19*(3), 1050. https://www.mdpi.com/1660-4601/19/3/1050

Fleming, R., & Bennett, K. (2015). Assessing the Quality of Environmental Design in Nursing Homes for People with Dementia: Development of a New Tool. *Australasian Journal on Aging*, *34*(3), 191–194. https://doi.org/10.1111/ajag.12233

Palm, R., Köhler, K., Bartholomeyczik, S., & Holle, B. (2014). Assessing the Application of Non-pharmacological Interventions for People with Dementia in German Nursing Homes: Feasibility and Content Validity of the Dementia Care Questionnaire (DemCare-Q). *BMC Research Notes*, *7*, 950. https://doi.org/10.1186/1756-0500-7-950

Project 2

Decision-making in care homes: the impact of the environment on people living with dementia sharing their everyday decisions

Rachel Daly

Introduction

Little is known about the part that people living with dementia and associated communication difficulties play in making and sharing decisions about their everyday life in care homes. The Person-Centred Practice Framework (McCormack & McCance, 2016) highlights the importance of effective relationships and shared power and decision-making in care environments. Sharing in everyday decision-making about, for example, their health and care is important to people living with dementia, but this is underestimated by care staff and families (Daly et al., 2018).

Experimental approach

This Appreciative Inquiry study engaged 15 people living with dementia, 24 care staff, and four family members in two care homes in England to explore how they make and share everyday decisions.

Appreciative Inquiry is useful for researching and stimulating change in social systems with its four interrelated stages: (1) Discovery, (2) Dream, (3) Design, and (4) Destiny (Cooperrider et al., 2008). Each stage relies on participants sharing their stories, ideas, and experiences. Appreciative Inquiry reflects the shared decision-making process between people living with dementia, care staff, and family care partners.

Modified Appreciative Inquiry approaches (Clouder & King, 2015) have previously been successfully employed in care home research (Amador et al., 2016). Here, we adapted it to combine the Discover and Dream stages, to reduce cognitive load and time pressures for participants. During 72 hours of observation, 13 focus groups and 26 interviews, participants demonstrated that people living with dementia and communication difficulties regularly make and share in 20 different everyday decisions.

Most effective shared decisions entailed simple choices related to food and drink, physical and social activities, and aspects of personal care. However,

DOI: 10.4324/9781003416241-23

some people also shared complex decisions with multiple care partners over extended time periods that relied on people knowing and understanding each other well. Maximising shared everyday decision-making depended on participants' effective use of six enabling factors: (1) Environment, (2) Encouragement, (3) Communication, (4) Choice, (5) Time, and (6) Identifying an appropriate decision partner (Daly, 2019).

In addition to understanding shared decision-making patterns, participants' contributed ideas to enhance shared everyday decision-making practice in their care homes. These included the presentation of food and everyday information in a more accessible manner (including pictures with words), and a post-box to increase written communications between residents and their care partners. The most popular idea was a shop inside the care home where residents would have choice and control over what they purchased and the opportunity to use money.

The care home environment as a decision-making enabler

The care home environment was found to enable shared everyday decision-making on macro, meso, and micro levels.

The macro-level was the physical setting (i.e., modern, spacious and light, encouraging interaction), using clear signage and simple, clutter free, décor along with a positive care home culture; and, in addition, (for some residents) accessible, safe outside spaces. There were inevitable environmental limitations on everyday decision-making; for example, freedom of movement due to locked doors, and meals and activities being limited to two or three choices.

Meso-levels of environmental facilitation included routines incorporating multiple residents' preferences. For example, care staff provided breakfast throughout the day for residents to take when and where they chose. Staff largely took the use of environmental adjustment to maximise residents' comfort and minimise distress for granted. It was undervalued, particularly by staff. In addition, medication times were incorporated into numerous residents' preferred care patterns.

Micro-level enablement was in positioning the person as capable. Participants living with dementia often discussed autonomy, although how they perceived it, varied. Staff facilitated so-called 'autonomous' decisions by clarifying options, manipulating environments, and creating choice. Care staff often communicated with residents using visual aids, gestures, and environmental modifications to compensate for dementia-related confusion and reduced concentration. This was done by using individualised signs, objects, or signals, giving the person a greater sense of control. For example, clothing was presented in a way that was more accessible for the individual to decide what to wear that day.

Table 17.1 Six critical enabling factors for shared everyday decision-making in care homes (above) and Example from observation notes (below)

Enabling factor	Key messages
Encouragement	Motivational support for a person living with dementia to do something that is considered to be in their best interest, or confidence to try something new.
Communication	Tailored multisensory approaches (e.g. simplifying language, breaking down compound decisions, using visual aids) to facilitate decision-making processes.
Choices	Choices are either (1) simplified by offering only two choices or (2) expanded by offering all available options with relevant information and advisory support.
Environment	Care home routines and physical environments are manipulated to facilitate multiple individual preferences and participation in decision-making.
Decision partner	The decision-making process (including who is involved) is shaped by the preferences of the person with dementia and the decision to be made.
Time	Time and space are provided to facilitate decision-making for people with fluctuating capacity and enable 'in-the-moment' decisions.
Example from observation notes	
	08.48 AM – We go to a female resident's room. Most people are still in bed, and we pass doors that are open but with residents still sleeping. The nurse explains that some residents must have medications at certain times, so they have to wake them, but most people wake up naturally and call when they want to get up. 'That's why we don't do the medication in room order.'

Conclusions

Care home environments can be effectively used to promote shared everyday decision-making with people living with dementia and communication difficulties on multiple levels (Table 17.1). Appreciative Inquiry promoted a high level of engagement, acknowledging the equal value of all stakeholders in contributing to the development and implementation of interventions to enhance shared everyday decision-making in the care environment.

In-depth box

- People living with dementia and their care partners participated throughout the study, from observations to interviews and focus groups. They found Appreciative Inquiry acceptable as a method of engagement and it reflected the shared decision-making process.

- Participants designed innovative, affordable, and sustainable ideas to enhance shared everyday decision-making in their homes.
- Care homes worked with people living with dementia and their care partners to embrace and implement environmental changes including routines, picture boards and menus and a post box to enhance communication.

Funding statement

This work presents independent research funded by the National Institute for Health Research (NIHR) for Applied Research Collaboration (ARC) East of England, at Cambridgeshire and Peterborough NHS Foundation Trust. The views expressed are those of the author(s) and not necessarily those of the NHS, the NIHR or the Department of Health and Social Care.

Ethics

Ethical approval reference number: 226515.

References

Amador S, Goodman C, Mathie E, Nicholson C. Evaluation of an Organisational Intervention to Promote Integrated Working between Health Services and Care Homes in the Delivery of End-of-Life Care for People with Dementia: Understanding the Change Process Using a Social Identity Approach. *International Journal of Integrated Care*. 2016 Jun 3, 16(2), 14. doi: 10.5334/ijic.2426. PMID: 27616969; PMCID: PMC5015557.

Clouder, D.L. and King, V. (2015) 'What Works? A Critique of Appreciative Inquiry as a Research Method/ology' in Jeroen Huisman and Malcolm Tight (Eds). *Theory and method in higher education research II* (Vol. 10, pp. 169–190). Bingley, UK: Emerald Group Publishing Limited. http://dx.doi.org/10.1108/S2056-375220150000001008

Cooperrider, D. L., Stavros, J. M., & Whitney, D. (2008). *The appreciative inquiry handbook: for leaders of change.* Berrett-Koehler Publishers.

Daly, R. L. (2019) Everyday Decisions in care homes: understanding and facilitating the involvement of people living with dementia and communication difficulties through appreciative inquiry. Unpublished.

Daly, R. L., Bunn, F., & Goodman, C. (2018). Shared decision-making for people living with dementia in extended care settings: a systematic review. *BMJ open*, 8(6).

McCormack, B., & McCance, T. (Eds.). (2016). *Person-centred practice in nursing and health care: theory and practice.* John Wiley & Sons.

Epilogue

Eef Hogervorst and Tri Budi Rahardjo

The reality of dementia care at home and in hospitals

Fleming and Zeisel (this volume) demonstrated that there is widespread agreement on the important principles supporting good design for people with dementia, and set out some of the important work they, and others, have carried out in order to advance their implementation. Here we present some of our experiences and observations across a number of countries and cultures relevant to both the progress and lack of progress in this field.

Best practice, but not affordable?

In 2021, Loughborough University was tendered to design a specialised dementia facility by a local council using principles of person-centred care as set out by Kitwood (1997). This approach has 7 core values: individuality, independence, privacy, partnership, choice, dignity, respect and rights. Difficult interactions between patients and care staff are seen as an expression of unmet needs, with difficulty in communicating such needs and receiving appropriate solutions to meet them. Person-centred care leads to improved quality of life for both carers and people with dementia, and better support and training for care staff using the person-centred approach in hospitals also led to substantial savings including retaining of staff, as Professor Clive Ballard's studies in the UK showed (Halsall, Riley, and Hogervorst, 2023).

Here, the established dementia inclusive design aspects derived from our work with the Chris and Sally house were employed (see Jain and Hogervorst, this volume) and again Bill Halsall's HLP group excelled in their designs. This was supported by many interviews with involved service users and service providers who had decided on person-centred design. Approaches promoted by Kevin Charras were incorporated. Open dining was used in the Loughborough/HLP dementia specialist facility design; enabling people to make their own food, come to eat at a large communal table and go when they wanted, engage in other activities in the communal space and navigate the spaces without hindrance. This approach struck a chord with all involved

DOI: 10.4324/9781003416241-24

and was implemented throughout in the specialist dementia facility design. Massage and touch were included in the specialist dementia facility plan, as these had a reasonable evidence base to suggest such treatments could calm people and improve their quality of life. Engagement with outdoor spaces, reminiscence activities, gardening, music and the arts, supported by local work also played an important role in the design of the facility.

However, sadly, the projected £7.5 m facility never happened. After two years of intense work (before which the council had worked on this project for 5 years to secure the best site, and have consultations, etc.), with conferences and workshops, with PPIE designers, architects and academics , there was no money for the actual build, and so the plans for the beautiful facility were unfortunately shelved.

Meanwhile, Loughborough was also asked by the burgeoning private sector to vet and research the 'dementia friendly' design of their care homes. The dull blues, creams and greys were not entirely au fait, as were the heavy ornaments which regularly destroyed the furniture when people's needs apparently were not met, but many features for activities were fine, for those who could afford it. As these companies would not pay for research and their design was a mere nod to some of the proposed dementia-friendly guidelines, further collaborative work was not pursued.

India: the importance of care staff

In Bangalore, India, Eef visited the Nightingale facility in 2012 which provided personalised care for people living there with dementia. It was simple: a bus stop in the closed large, beautiful garden for anxious people who wanted to go home, but ultimately ended up getting distracted by passers-by, butterflies, birds, or their appetite, which made them wander back inside. The agitated man who would be called by a nurse pretending to be his daughter who had passed away. An angry man who would be calmed with his favourite records played. All this information about each patient was noted down on large sheets hanging behind the beds.

Some of this care might be considered by Kitwood (1997) as typical of malignant social psychology, undermining personhood of people living with dementia (via treachery, withholding, invalidation, disempowerment, etc.). This type of care would thus not be considered person-centred (Mitchell and Agnelli, 2015). Still, it was done with kindness, calmness and respect and avoided confrontation and frustration. Importantly, medication to calm people was used minimally using these almost playful personalised distraction approaches. There was a multi-sensory room, and various activities were organised, but people could choose whether they wanted to attend or engage in their own preferred activities. Each three patients had one trained carer keeping an eye on them and to engage with them as a family member. These carers were people from the poorer parts of the town, who had been trained in care onsite and did this care in return for daily meals and a small stipend.

End of life in the Netherlands

The person-centred approach does not always tally with the regimented time-tables and schemas for the much-pressured care staff in hospitals, leaving very little time for personal needs, wants and the agendas of service users. Existing care policies can also interfere with such person-centred care. Often-times, there is a dissonance between what good, person-centred care should be, and what it ends up being. For instance, Eef's personal experience accompanying her mum in her final weeks in 2022 in the Netherlands was a far cry from both medical and person-centred guidelines. With a delirium, due to not identified heart failure despite repeated calls to her GP, Eef's mum was diagnosed with dementia at a memory clinic. Neither blood tests nor physical examinations were carried out. She was then moved twice, as the hospitals which had beds available, could not admit people with dementia due to policies.

Untreated severe constipation and gum infection that caused difficulty eating and a severe lack of nutrition were suspected to contribute to the cognitive impairment and confusion, but were not examined or treated by any of the hospital staff, despite urging from the family to do so. In the final dementia-friendly hospital, many miles from home, after assessment, the medical team decided she had to go to a closed dementia ward, as there was no space in any of the (few remaining) care homes. The reason given for moving her in such a poor state was to keep mortality rates of the hospital low, and there was no space at a hospice to die either. She was also not allowed to be discharged home, and no private carers were available for many weeks. A claim against the hospital was filed by a personal care worker and while waiting, Eef's mum (always the rebel) died peacefully on her own terms in the beautiful very dementia inclusive ward.

The importance of people vs technology in dementia care

In 2010, Eef visited an old Indonesian, former Dutch colonial psychiatric hospital. She was hosted at the Dr Rajiman Wediodiningrat State Mental Health Hospital in Lawang-Malang East Java Indonesia by Dr Yuniar Sunarko, a specialist old-age psychiatrist. The museum showed some of the horrible practices that were used in the colonial past, such as a lukewarm bath where people stayed in for days, a medieval-looking electroshock treatment and tight swaddling. In sharp contrast, the current Indonesian staff had implemented all the ideas they had picked up from dementia-friendly design. There was good contrast between floors and walls, and railings were on every wall to provide support for people and reduce risk of falls. People were guarded closely to avoid slips and falls when floors were mopped. They helped to cook the meals and engage in other reminiscence activities with youngsters to teach them old crafts, music-making and storytelling. Signs helped for orientation in time and place. There was dancing and singing, while sheep and bunnies hopped around for pet therapy, ignorant of any health and safety regulations. With many staff present, falls were very rare, and people had little need for calming medication.

In the beautiful, multi-million (but largely empty) dementia-friendly hospital Eef visited in the Netherlands in 2022 to be present for her mum's final weeks, there were expensive technology-supported activity tools and gym equipment on every green marble clad industrial designed floor. None of these were ever seen to be used. The tablets provided per bed to use the television, music, curtains and lights were too complicated for most older people, and certainly for those with dementia and/or confusion. The staff were too busy to help, with buttons to press mostly ignored, leaving most people lying lonely in their beds staring at the walls. When people cried out in pain, anger or fear, they were usually ignored. With fewer people wanting to work in the care sector with its sometimes-brutal decision-making and high-pressured environments, the question is whether technology could support design to (a) keep older people in their homes and (b) alleviate some of the care burden of professional carers in the hospital and care homes.

It must be kept in mind that Eef's visits to India and Indonesia described above were done more than a decade ago and those care facilities will all have changed with the times. This agility of these homes, which had at the time implemented dementia inclusive aspects quickly and cheaply, was impressive. But the numbers of people, the staff, who contributed to providing this level of kind and personalised care was also very large. We are a social species, and loneliness is one of the largest risk factors for dementia (Irving et al., 2018). The milk of human kindness, to belong and interact with others, is crucial for our health. Isolating a human is the worst punishment we can give. Can the human touch be replaced by a robot? Technology also often breaks down, as even seen with simple scanning technology encountered in supermarkets and at airports.

Where technology did seem to work was in Japan, when Eef briefly visited hospitals and care homes in 2010, and where there was a strong emphasis on rehabilitation and keeping older people active. However, appropriate engagement with such technology still requires trained staff. With Japan's ageing population, the more formal approach culturally required in such care, however, did not support nursing staff migration from some other countries. The formality needed there was counter to the warm, kind and personable approach found in the Indonesian care staff, for instance. This type of ethnic migration is more commonly seen to fill these undervalued care positions, but can be difficult with language and cultural barriers. It is also unethical, given the much lower pay this type of staff often receive, while being displaced away from family and often children, which can create stress, heartache, homesickness and poor health in these carers. A recent article in *The Guardian* likened the treatment of these 'imported' care home and private residency staff to modern slavery (Booth, 2024)

With increasing inflation and costs of living, Brexit and several wars, there is now also a large proportion of very poor people in the UK who cannot eat or heat their houses. Should care homes provide them food and heat so they provide community support for older people with dementia, as was done in India and Indonesia?

The way forward: a change of heart is needed

Perhaps as a society, we have to decide whether the private market can take care of the sick, the dying, of health, education and welfare. With the gap between the rich and poor growing faster in the last twenty years than it has in a long time, we all need to evaluate whether this is justified in any way and is appropriate for our level of civilisation. Perhaps a fairer society, where care of the old, our children, and the sick, is appropriately paid for, appreciated and commended can instead be the way forward.

A true person-centred approach where the needs of people with dementia are recognised is required and can save us all money. Giving people comfort (the feeling you can trust others); attachment (feeling secure and finding familiarity); inclusion and occupation (being involved in the lives of others and in your own activities of daily living, such as making food) and identity (being recognised as an individual) are core needs (Mitchell and Agnelli, 2015). We are not an individual species, we thrive on love, compassion, and connection. The design of our homes and environments should reflect these needs and this should include the people designed for from the start, but also those who care, to be appreciated financially and societally by us all.

In depth box

- Person-centred design can improve the quality of life of staff and of people living with dementia, as well as save costs due to lower need for medical specialist interventions.
- However, technology and other expensive solutions by themselves are not always the best answers to meet needs if these are not supported by trained and kind staff. Better financial and societal appreciation of care staff is imperative to ensure optimal quality of life for people living with dementia.

References

Booth, R. 2024. Modern slavery in social care surging since visa rules eased. https://www.theguardian.com/society/2024/jan/21/modern-slavery-in -social-care-surging-since-visa-rules-eased (accessed 23 Jan 2024).

Halsall, B., Riley, M., & Hogervorst, E., 2023. *Design for dementia: living well at home*. Routledge: London.

Irving, K., Hogervorst, E., Oliveira, D., Kivipelto, & M, editors., 2018. *New developments in dementia prevention research: state of the art and future possibilities*. Routledge: London UK.

Kitwood, T, 1997. *Dementia reconsidered: the person comes first*. Open University Press: Buckingham.

Mitchell, G., & Agnelli, J. 2015. Person-centred care for people with dementia: Kitwood reconsidered. *Nursing standard (Royal College of Nursing (Great Britain): 1987)*, 30(7), 46–50. https://doi.org/10.7748/ns.30.7.46.s47

Index

Note: **Bold** page numbers refer to tables; *italic* page numbers refer to figures and page numbers followed by "n" denote endnotes.

ACQSC *see* Australian Aged Care Quality and Safety Commission (ACQSC)
activity 4, 33, 61, 83, 89, 150, 184, 207, 227; meaningful 150, 172, 187, 189, 206, 209
AD *see* Alzheimer's disease (AD)
ADI *see* Alzheimer's Disease International (ADI)
adult day services (ADSs) 205, 206
age-friendly communities 109
aging 20, 22, 69, 109, 121, 125, 145, 157, 196–197, 200, 201, 227
AJDC *see* Australian Journal of Dementia Care (AJDC)
Aladawi, A. 24
Albayrak, A. 24
Alzheimer, A. 15
Alzheimer's disease (AD) 15–16, 20; CERAD criteria for 16; medical factors, assessment of 21
Alzheimer's Disease International (ADI) 6, 59, 173
architectural/architecture 49, 59, 69, 70, 73–76, 174, 175, 197, 199, 200; barriers 71; conventional communication tools and methods 72; dementia-sensitive 98–100; design process 71; evidence-based 46–47; guidance for general hospitals 157–166; health research 95–105; human needs in 104; models 45–46; residential care 47–48, *48*, *50*, 50–52
artificial intelligence 20, 211

Australasian Health Facility Guidelines 177
Australian Aged Care Quality and Safety Commission (ACQSC) 177, 180
Australian Journal of Dementia Care (AJDC) 174
Automatic Number Plate Recognition 113
autonomy 20, 34, 37, 39–41, 48, 49, 57, 59, 66, 120, 172, 187, 188, 196–201, 206, 209–211, 221

Ballard, C. 25
BEAT-D *see* Built Environment Audit Tool-Dementia (BEAT-D)
Begde, A. 24
Behavioural and Psychological Symptoms associated with Dementia (BPSD) 17, 21
Bennett, K. 172
BIM *see* building information modelling (BIM)
Bohnsack, R. 96
Bowes, A. 58
BPSD *see* Behavioural and Psychological Symptoms associated with Dementia (BPSD)
brain reserve capacity 18–19
British Standards Institute (BSI) 122
Brooker, D. 147
Brorsson, A. 96
BSI *see* British Standards Institute (BSI)
building information modelling (BIM) 72

built environment 6, 47, 57, 59, 61, 70, 74, 98, 104, 131, 132, 135, 137–140, 159, 174, 175, 177, 197, 208, 216, 217, 219; neighbourhood 61, 132–135; *see also* neighbourhood-built environment (NBE)
Built Environment Audit Tool-Dementia (BEAT-D) 176
Burgstaller, M. 147
Büter, K. 98
Byers, S. 46

CAD *see* computer aided design (CAD)
C.A.D.E. (Confused and Disturbed Elderly) units 32, 37–38
Calkins, M. P. 45, 172
Cammen, T. van der 24
caregivers 49–52, 82–86, 89, 90, 95, 96, 98, 100, 103–104, 161, 199, 200, 205–209
care homes 2, 3, 8, 9, 20, 21, 23–25, 30–41, 52, 58, 84, 120, 121, 127, 129, 131, 195–201, 225–228; decision-making in 220–223; environment framework 208–209; ethics of care 49; farming 205–207; Nightingale care home 25
care-receiving 51
care tools 25
Carlson, L. A. 195
Carp, F. M. 32
Carpman, J. R. 195
Chappell, N. L. 148
citizenship 6
co-creation 208, 210, 211
co-design 7, 24, 58, 66, 69, 70, 73, 74, 77, 82–90, 152; with dementia experts by lived experience 60–62; feedback on 87–88; prototype solutions, developing and delivering 86–87, *87*, *88*
cognitive psychology 195–196
cognitive reserve capacity 18–19
cognitive spectrum disorders 146
Cohen, U. 34, 37, 45, 172; *Contemporary Environments for People with Dementia* 33; design principles **35–36**; *Holding on to Home* 33
comfort 31, 49, 61, 74, 189, 221, 228
community care 3, 208
community engagement 110–111

Competence-Press Model *see* environment(al), Docility Hypothesis
computer aided design (CAD) 72
Contemporary Environments for People with Dementia (Cohen and Day) 33
Cook, M. 23, 24
Coons, D. 32
COORDINATES project 83
co-production 75; *see also* co-design
co-researchers 119, 125, 138, 208
Corinne Dolan Center 37
CRPD *see* United Nations Convention on the Rights of Persons with Disabilities 2006 (CRPD)
culture: and dementia 18; lifestyle 78n4

DAI *see* Dementia Alliance International (DAI)
Davis, S. 46
Dawson, A. 58
Day, K. 37; *Contemporary Environments for People with Dementia* 33; design principles **35–36**
day care centres 98
DDM *see* Double Diamond Model (DDM)
decision-making, in care homes 220–223, **222**
DEEP (Dementia Engagement and Empowerment Project) 122
De Hogeweyk/Hogewey Dementia Village, The Netherlands 40
delirium 22–23, 226; delirium superimposed on dementia (DSD) 146
dementia: culture and 18; design as prevention of progression to dependency 19–20; design to promote mental health 19–20; diagnosis, reliability of 23; as disease with characteristic pathology 15; frontotemporal 17–18; Lewy body 17–18; medical factors, assessment of 21–22; onset of 21–22; Parkinson's disease 17–18; prevention of 15; symptoms, progression of 18–19; vascular 16–17; *see also individual entries*
Dementia Alliance International (DAI) 39; Environmental Design Special Interest Group 59–60
Dementia Care Mapping 5

Dementia Centre 122
Dementia Design Assessment Tool 70
Dementia Friendly Communities (DFC)
    59, 62
dementia-friendly hospitals (DFHs)
    145–153; characterising 148;
    experiences of 146–148; guidelines
    and self-assessment, role of 151–152;
    outcomes of 146; practices and
    policies, evaluation of 149–150;
    provider perspective on 150–151
"Dementia-friendly Library Wiener
    Neustadt, The" 96, 100–102,
    101, 102
dementia rights, designing for
    58–59
dementia-sensitive architecture:
    implementation in public buildings
    99–100; principles of 98–99
Dementia Training Australia 174, 175,
    177
Demonstrating Impact in Housing,
    Health and Social Care (DIHHSC)
    69, 73–74, 76
DemSCAPE project 61, 62
"DEN-HB – Dementia-Enabling
    Neighbourhoods: Participatory
    Development of Dementia-Friendly
    Neighbourhoods in Bremen" 132–
    135, *134*
Department of Health New South Wales
    Report, Australia (1983) 32
DesHCA *see* Designing Homes for
    Health Cognitive Ageing (DesHCA)
design 195–201; checklists 5, 10;
    co-design 7, 24, 58, 60–63, 66, 69,
    70, 73, 74, 77, 82–90, 152; inclusive
    15–26, 72, 104, 119–129, 174, 224;
    universal 152
'Design, dignity, dementia:
    dementia-related design and the built
    environment' (2020 World Alzheimer
    Report) 6, 39, 40, 59, 132, 173
Design Dignity Manifesto 173, 175
Design for Dementia (Judd) 33
*Design for Dementia: Planning
    Environments for the Elderly and
    Confused* (Calkins) 32–33
Designing Homes for Health Cognitive
    Ageing (DesHCA) 69, 74–76
DFC *see* Dementia Friendly
    Communities (DFC)

DFHs *see* dementia-friendly hospitals
    (DFHs)
dignity 6, 39, 57, 59, 83, 109, 120, 128,
    209, 210
DIHHSC *see* Demonstrating Impact
    in Housing, Health and Social Care
    (DIHHSC)
distress/distressing/distressed 34, 64, 82,
    114, 121, 125, 127, 147; emotional
    distress in using 124–125
DMT *see* Dunhill Medical Trust (DMT)
domus philosophy 4, 9
Double Diamond Model (DDM) 83, *83*
DSD *see* delirium superimposed on
    dementia (DSD)
Duah-Owusu White, M. 150
Dunhill Medical Trust (DMT) 19, 24
Dunn, B. B. 19

EAT-HC *see* Environmental Audit
    Tool – High Care (EAT-HC)
Economic and Social Research Council
    (ESRC) 20
Edinburgh Centre for Research on the
    Experience of Dementia (ECRED)
    122
EDSiG *see* Environmental Design
    Special Interest Group (EDSiG)
Egan, J. 72
EHE *see* 'Enhancing the Healing
    Environment' (EHE) initiative
elderly mentally infirm (EMI) homes 2
empower/empowerment 6, 48, 49, 103;
    disempower 20, 147, 225; *see also*
    co-design; co-production
end of life, in the Netherlands 226
'Enhancing the Healing Environment'
    (EHE) initiative 6, 70, 151
environment(al): accessible environment
    60; built 6, 47, 57, 59, 61, 70, 74,
    98, 104, 131, 132, 135, 137–140,
    159, 174, 175, 177, 197, 208,
    216, 217, 219; court 64, 66; design
    development 57–58; design for
    dementia 70–71; design knowledge
    into practice 171–180; Design
    Service 175; Docility Hypothesis 31;
    press 31; psychology 195–196
Environmental Audit Tool – High Care
    (EAT-HC) 217–219
Environmental Design Special Interest
    Group (EDSiG) 59–60

environment characteristics: comfort 31,
49, 61, 74, 189, 221, 228; homelike
33, 34, 35, 37, 41, 58, 172, 198,
207, 209–210; homeliness 2, 4, 5,
9, 10; household 34, 37, 38, 40, 41,
209, 210; privacy 5, 25, 37, 40, 147,
160, 172, 187, 224
equality 47, 49
Equality Act 2010 (UK) 128
equity 47–49
ergonomic agricultural design model 45;
see also green care farms
ESRC *see* Economic and Social Research
Council (ESRC)
European Working Group of People
with Dementia 109–110
evidence-based architectural design
46–47
EVOLVE 199
experiential agricultural design model
46
Eynard, C. 46, 49

family involvement 4, 9, 187, 190
"Find Your Way" project 62–64, 65
flooring 103, 124, 149, 151
Focus on Dementia Network 110
Friendship House of Cedar Lake Home
37
frontotemporal dementia 17–18

G-EAT *see* German Environmental
Audit Tool (G-EAT)
Geller Institute of Ageing and Memory
120
general hospitals 5, 8–9; architectural
design guidance for 157–166;
dementia-friendly emergency
departments, requirements of
160–162, *161*, *162*; future designs,
directions for 163–165; spatial
anchor points in wards 162–163,
164; into urban environments,
integration of 159–160
German Alzheimer's Society 157–158
German Environmental Audit Tool
(G-EAT) 70, 175, 199, 217–219
Grant, M. A. 195
green care farms 8, 40, 205–211
Green House Project™ 40
Grey, T. 152

Halsall, B. 24
HammondCare 122

Haslam, N.: *Psychology in the
Bathroom* 119
Hawkins, R. 174
healing 47–49
Hiatt, L. G. 32, 45
*Hidden no more. Dementia and
disability* report (UK All Party Group
Parliamentary on Dementia) 128
Hignett, S. 23
Holding on to Home (Cohen and
Weisman) 33
homely/homelike/homeliness, care
environment 2, 4, 9, 33, 34, 37, 41,
58, 172, 198, 207, 209–210, 224
homeostasis 31
hospitalization, of people with dementia
157–158
Houghton, C. 147
housing decisions, improving 82–90
human–environment interaction:
behaviour 15–18, 21–23, 25, 57, 58,
70, 77, 119, 121, 145, 148–150, 157,
159, 160, 172, 184, 189, 195, 197,
198, 200, 201, 208; experience 146–
148; orientation 3, 10, 16, 21, 24,
34, 46, 96–100, 103, 113, 114, 131,
135, 137, 139, 140, 147, 149, 150,
158–160, 162, 172, 186, 188, 197–
201, 227; Person–Environment (P–E)
interaction 46; wayfinding 8, 21, 32,
34, 62–64, 65, 98, 99, 114, 131–133,
137–140, 147, 150, 151, 195–201
human rights 9, 49, 59, 60, 66, 119,
122, 128, 211
Hyde, J. 45

INCLUDE 137, 139, 140
inclusivity/inclusion 9, 15–26,
47–49, 137–140; accessibility 72;
dementia-free 137–140; usability 76
India, importance of care staff in 225
indoor environments 24, 97, 99, 195,
200, 201, 208
innovation 8, 30, 31, 34, 39–41, 51,
111, 114, 115, 131, 132, 135, 163,
165, 175, 176, 205–211
institutional environment 1, 2, 9
integration 2, 9, 158, 159
INTERDEM 7, 25
involvement: co-creation 208; co-design
62, 66; consultation 51, 74;
co-production 75, 78; co-research
140; engagement 4, 24, 62, 110, 114;
patient and public involvement 24

Jais, C. 23
Judd, S. 38; *Design for Dementia* 33;
    design principles **35–36**

Kamp, D. 174
Karr, J.-B. A. 41
Kelly, F. 150
key themes, discovering and defining
    84–86, **84–85**
Kidd, B. 37
King's Fund, The 3, 151
Kirch, J. 151
KITE project 61
Kitwood, T. 4, 5, 25, 49, 189, 225
Koch, S. 46
Koos Service Design 84

Latham, M. 72
Lawton, M. P. 30, 31, 45, 172
Levkoff, S. 45
Lewy body dementia 17–18
lifestyle 16, 17, 78n4, 209
Lindsay, S. 89
long-term care 2, 4, 5, 30, 32, 45, 46,
    70, 98, 171, 184–192, 196, 199–201,
    207–211, 217

Mace, N.: *36 Hour Day* 32
Manietta, C. 148
Marshall, M. 45, 172
Massive Open Online Courses
    (MOOCs) 174
Masterson, A. 151
McDonnell, R. 24
McKeith, I. G. 17
Memory Care Assisted Living
    Communities 174
Mini Mental State Examination
    (MMSE) 18
mixed-methods design 61
MMSE *see* Mini Mental State
    Examination (MMSE)
mobility 99, 101, 102, 104, 122, 187
MOOCs *see* Massive Open Online
    Courses (MOOCs)
Morgan, D. G. 46
Moss, B. 37

Nahemow, L. 31
National Aged Care Design Principles
    and Guidelines 180
National Dementia Plans 7, 171, 180
National Dementia Strategy, England
    151

National Health Service (NHS) 2, 4, 5
natural environment 60
navigation 19, 99, 137, 139, 140, 160,
    162, 195, 196, 198–200, 201
Nay, R. 46
NBE *see* neighbourhood-built
    environment (NBE)
NCSD *see* non-cognitive symptoms of
    dementia (NCSD)
needs-based agricultural design model
    46; *see also* green care farms
neighbourhood-built environment
    (NBE) 61, 132–135; criteria **133**;
    experimental approach 132–133;
    preliminary results 133–134
New South Wales Health 177
NHS *see* National Health Service (NHS)
non-cognitive symptoms of dementia
    (NCSD) 146, 147
normalisation 3, 9
nursing homes 30, 32, 37, 45, 98,
    120, 158, 186, 205, 206, 210, 211;
    German environmental audit tool in
    217–223

"opportunities for meaningful
    wandering" 33, 34
organisational environment 188, 190,
    191, 208–209
othering 71–72
orientation 96–97; aids 3, 10; human–
    environment interaction 3, 10, 16,
    21, 24, 34, 46, 96–100, 103, 113,
    114, 131, 135, 137, 139, 140, 147,
    149, 150, 158–160, 162, 172, 186,
    188, 197–201, 227; individual 97;
    social 96, 97
outdoor: environment 5, 34, 40, 61,
    96–97, 120, 172, 195, 206, 208;
    mobility 96–97
overstimulation 31
Oxford Project to Investigate Memory
    and Ageing 22

PAMIS (Promoting a more inclusive
    society) 122
Parke, B. 148
Parkinson's dementia 17–18
participation 37, 58, 60–62, 72, 73, 78,
    82, 95, 96, 100, 103–105, 109, 128,
    186, 192, 206, 211
participatory design process 69–78; *see
    also* co-design

Patient and Public Involvement and Engagement (PPPIE) 24
PBSD *see* psychological behavioural symptoms of dementia (PBSD)
PCC *see* person-centred care (PCC)
people *vs.* technology, in dementia care 226–228
personalised designing 25
person-centered goals 34
person-centred care (PCC) 4, 5, 10, 49, 146, 151, 189, 190, 211, 224, 226
person-centred design 6, 7, 25, 224, 228
PhotoVoice Hamilton 122
physical environment 2, 5, 6, 8–10, 95, 104, 105, 146, 149, 150–152, 188, 190–192, 197, 199, 200, 208–210
PLAN-ACT-OBSERVE-REFLECT cycle 189
PLAN-EAT 176
PPPIE *see* Patient and Public Involvement and Engagement (PPPIE)
practice: dementia-friendly hospitals 149–150; environmental design knowledge into practice, translation of 171–180
privacy 5, 25, 37, 40, 147, 160, 172, 187, 224
proof of care 50–52, *50*
prosthetic environment 3
prototype solutions, developing and delivering 86–87, **87**, *88*
Psychogeriatric Rating Scale 38
psychological behavioural symptoms of dementia (PBSD) 70; *see also* Behavioural and Psychological Symptoms associated with Dementia (BPSD)
Psychology in the Bathroom (Haslam) 119
psychosocial environment 146
public buildings and services 95–105
public organizations: dementia-sensitive 95–96, 100–105
public spaces 102–103
public toilets 62–63
public transport 102–103
Purandare, N. 45

quality of life 5, 6, 15, 25, 46, 57, 59, 60, **85**, 109, 128, 159, 184, 187–192, 196, 210, 224, 225, 228

Rabins, P. V.: *36 Hour Day* 32
Reality Orientation (RO) 3

Regnier, V. 174
rehabilitative agricultural design model 45
rehabilitative environment 60
Reilly, J. C. 147
reminiscence 3, 10, 225, 227
research methods: co-design 7, 24, 58, 60–64, 66, 69, 70, 73, 74, 77, 82–90, 152; co-research 137–140; participatory action research 115, 137, 138, 140; qualitative 47, 96, 133, 137; quantitative 47; real world 52; virtual reality 69–78; walking interviews 96, 100, 101, 105, 109, 138, 218
reserve capacity 18–19
residential care: architectural design 47–48, *48*, *50*, 50–52; environments 47–48, *48*, *50*, 50–52, 195–201; homes, minimizing spatial disorientation in 195–201; homes, navigability of 199–200; residential care homes 195–201
Residential Care Home Navigability scale 199
rights 3, 9; right to self-determination 39; United Nations Convention on the Rights of Persons with Disabilities 2006 (CRPD) 59, 128
RO *see* Reality Orientation (RO)
Roberts, B. 24
Royal Melbourne Institute of Technology (RMIT University) 175
rural environments 109–115

Sanders, E. B. N. 89
SBS Transit 62
SCUs *see* Special Care Units (SCUs)
segregation 2, 9, 30, 59
self-advocacy 76, 135
self-esteem 83, 189
sensory deprivation 31
sensory stimulation 33, 58
signage 6, 34, 64, 100, 101, 114, 120, 123, 126, 127, 133, 147, 149, 163, 172, 195, 197–201, 221
social care 2, 86, 206
social environment 2, 5, 8–10, 59, 95, 103–105, 131, 147, 184, 188, 190–192, 208, 209, 219
social orientation 96, 97
sociotherapeutic living environments (STLs): action research 189–191; central aspects **185**; general

considerations 190–191; in long-term care organisations 184–192; practice documentation 186–187; problem statement 184–186; published studies 187–188, *188*; recommendations for 191–192; research area 184–186; for residents with dementia and person-centred care 189
Special Care Units (SCUs) 30
Stappers, P. J. 89
Stewart, N. J. 46
STLs *see* sociotherapeutic living environments (STLs)
sustainable environment 60

taking care 51
technology in the environment 60
therapeutic agricultural design model 45
Therapeutic Environmental Screening Survey 70
36 Hour Day (Mace & Rabins) 32
Thomas, B. 174
toilets 6, 8, *62–63*, 101, *102*, 103, 119–129; finding 126–127; positioning of 127; public inconvenience 121–126, **123**, *124*, *125*; public toilet 63, 103, 119, 121, 123–125; refurbishment of-120
traditional medical model 15; benefits of 20
transportation 60, 96, 102–103; Accessible Travel Framework, Scotland 122; cognitive inclusivity 112–113; digitalisation in 112–113; future of 114; rural 109–115; technology in 110–111; and travel 60, 96, 102–103, 109–115; urban 109–115Try Before You Ride initiatives 114

vascular dementia (VaD) 16–17
Viatour, G. 46, 49
'VIPS' framework (Values, Individualised approach, Perspective of person with dementia, Social environment) 147
virtual reality (VR) 69–78; barriers to engagement, removing 75–76; co-production 75; and digital technology opportunities 73; experimental approach 73–75, *73*; implications on environmental design 77; remote engagement 76–77; wider inclusion 76–77

Waller, S. 151
wandering 34, 38
Wang, G. 24, 25
wayfinding 8, 21, 32, 34, 62–64, *65*, 98, 99, 114, 131–133, 137–140, 147, 150, 151, 195–201
Weisman, G. D. 45, 172
Weisman, J. 34; design principles **35–36**; *Holding on to Home* 33
Weiss Pavilion, Philadelphia Geriatric Center 31, 32, 37
well-being 5, 6, 38, 48, 50, 58, 66, 82, 98, 121, 158, 159, 166, 171, 184, 196, 197, 199–201; care farming, impact of 205–207; emotional 207; mental 186; physical 186; resident 41; social 189, 190, 192; staff 41
Woodside Place 37
World Health Organization 59

For Product Safety Concerns and Information please contact our
EU representative GPSR@taylorandfrancis.com Taylor & Francis
Verlag GmbH, Kaufingerstraße 24, 80331 München, Germany